Laparoscopic Liver Resection

Rong Liu

Laparoscopic Liver Resection

Theory and Techniques

Springer

Rong Liu
Surgical Oncology
Chinese PLA General Hospital
Beijing, China

ISBN 978-94-017-9734-4 ISBN 978-94-017-9735-1 (eBook)
https://doi.org/10.1007/978-94-017-9735-1

Library of Congress Control Number: 2017953440

Printed on acid-free paper

This Springer imprint is published by Springer Nature
The registered company is Springer Science+Business Media B.V.
The registered company address is: Van Godewijckstraat 30, 3311 GX Dordrecht, The Netherlands

Preface

Since the first laparoscopic cholecystectomy was performed in 1987, almost 30 years have elapsed. Although laparoscopic technique had been gradually applied in almost every area of surgery, laparoscopic liver resection (LLR) underwent a slow development all over the world since the first case was performed in 1991, especially in the first decade, mainly due to sophisticated anatomy, risk of bleeding, lack of ideal instrument, and concern for adequate margins in resection of malignant tumors. As a result, there were only a few cases of LLR performed, most of which were resections of solid tumor limited in the left lateral section or the margins and cystic fenestration, and the feasibility and efficiency of LLR had been questioned.

We have been performing LLR since 2001 and reported the first case of laparoscopic hemihepatectomy, laparoscopic right trisegmentectomy, laparoscopic modeling left lateral sectionectomy, single-incision laparoscopic liver resection, and retroperitoneal laparoscopic liver resection in China or all over the world. Based on those experiences, we established our unique technique and theory system of anatomic laparoscopic liver resection, which is characterized by precontrol of the blood supply of the to-be-resected area and prevention of bleeding, and have performed over 1000 cases of laparoscopic liver resection to date.

Benefiting from technique development and experience accumulation, in the recent 10 years, the application of minimally invasive technique in hepato-pancreato-biliary surgery had underwent rapid development, and LLR has been generally accepted after the Louisville Statement was announced in 2008. According to the literature, more than 3000 cases of LLR have been reported worldwide by 2014, and 50% of them were applied for malignant lesions. Not only the number of LLRs but also the ratio of major liver resections increased, and LLR for lesions in every segment was reported. The location of lesions was no longer considered as a contradiction for LLR anymore, and it was generally accepted that minimally invasive surgery has advantages such as smaller local trauma, milder systemic reactions, less operative blood loss, shorter hospital stay, lower morbidity, and better cosmetic results.

Despite all the achievements above, minimally invasive surgery is still not the majority of operations in hepato-pancreato-biliary surgery until now, not only in China but all over the world, and the technique varies from center to center, leading to difficulty in popularization. Thus, based on the experience of our LLR cases and the modeling or stylized surgery idea, we wrote this book, with plenty of pictures that demonstrate the operative and technical details presented, hopefully, to serve as reference and thus facilitate other centers to perform minimally invasive surgery.

As the first English book of our team, we do know that there are still some limitations of this book, and we are more than glad to receive judgments from peers all over the world, to make this book better and benefit more patients. Also, we will publish books focusing on laparoscopic pancreatectomy and robotic hepato-pancreato-biliary surgery, which will overcome the known difficulties during writing this book and hopefully be better.

On behalf of all the surgeons in our team, I would like to express my sincere acknowledgment to Academician Wu Mengchao and Academician Huang Zhiqiang, who are my mentors and had been supporting and guiding our team to perform minimally invasive surgery. We also would like to thank all the colleagues from the Department of Anesthesiology, Department of Nursing, Department of Intensive Care Unit, Department of Radiology, and so on, who helped us a lot to perform the surgeries. And thanks to all the patients, for trusting us and for being supportive to our writings.

Beijing, China Rong Liu

Contents

Laparoscopic Anatomical Hepatectomy

1

Abstract

Over the past 20 years, laparoscopic liver resection (LLR) has gone through a stirring process of innovation, development, and exploration. LLR nowadays is almost as important as OLR,. As an evolving surgical technique, LLR has its own inherent problems too. Laparoscopic anatomical hepatectomy (LAH), instead of laparoscopic regular hepatectomy, according to our experience, stands for the laparoscopic regional resection of hepatic tumor or hepatic segment(s), based on the regional control of blood supply. In this chapter, we will discuss what is LAH, its advantages and disadvantages and some key techniques.

Over the past 20 years, laparoscopic liver resection (LLR) has gone through a stirring process of innovation, development, and exploration (Fig. 1.1). In some resections (e.g., hepatic left lateral lobectomy), LLR is even expected to replace open liver resection (OLR) to become the gold standard procedure, just as laparoscopic cholecystectomy once did (Chang et al. 2007). Upon the whole, LLR nowadays is almost as important as OLR, with obvious superiorities including less blood loss and shorter length of hospital stay.

According to our experience, there are three key factors worthy of more attention in current practices: appropriate selection of indications and patients, full understanding of surgical instruments, and standardization of the procedure (Dagher et al. 2009).

As an evolving surgical technique, LLR has its own inherent problems even with the impressive improvement in the instruments and clinical experience. The wholly new surgical perspectives, pneumoperitoneum environment, special operative instruments, and other features together indicate that LLR might have its unique regularities different from those of OLR. The surgical experience of performing OLR can not help the surgeons to perform LLR directly. In some cases, the shackle of the old concept in OLR might lead to disastrous consequences in LLR. It is reasonable to adopt more stringent indications in LLR than in OLR. The size and

R. Liu, *Laparoscopic Liver Resection*,
https://doi.org/10.1007/978-94-017-9735-1_1

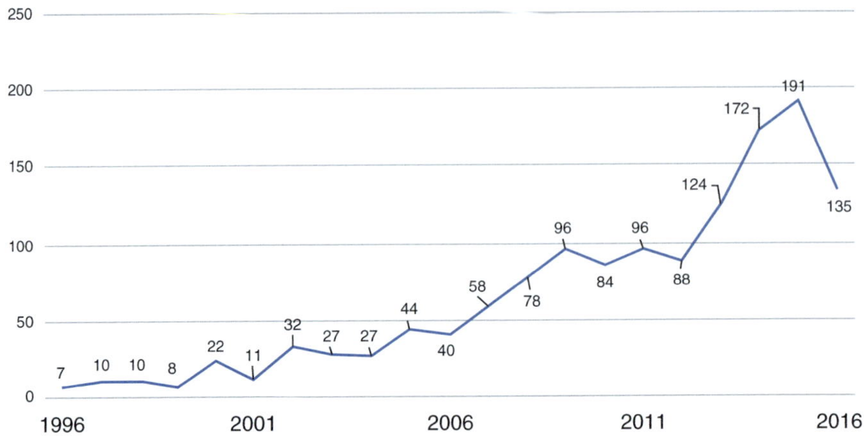

Fig. 1.1 The dramatically increased number of literatures about LLR

location of a liver tumor, and its spatial relationship with the liver hilum, major hepatic vessels and inferior vena cava, should be carefully reviewed before surgery. If a clear transection plane can be determined laparoscopically, LLR is preferred. Tumor size alone has not been the contraindication of LLR anymore. However, the choice between LLR and OLR should not change the consequent size of resection distinctly. Laparoscopic right hepatectomy resection is relatively easier than right posterior sectionectomy (Segments 6+7). If right posterior sectionectomy is sufficient for the lesion, open surgery should be adopted rather than laparoscopic right hepatectomy resection.

The newly published international consensus has given a panoramic understanding of this issue (Wakabayashi et al. 2015). Due to the lack of the tactile sensation, the cutting planes of liver resection were mainly determined by the preoperative imaging, landmark of the liver, and intraoperative navigation, rather than the hands of surgeons. Just like two sides of a coin, theoretically, LLR has advantages in surgical oncology for its essence of "no-touch" techniques. The full assessment of its surgical and oncological long-dated outcomes is still in progress. On the other hand, the advanced surgical instruments have played a much more important role in LLR than OLR. OLR could be performed using the simple crush-clamp technique without any energy device. The whole history of LLR has progressed on the basis of improvement of various energy equipments and stapling apparatuses. Laparoscopic surgeons must have full knowledge of the strength and limitations of tools available. This is the key to give full play to the devices and to avoid any unwanted complication.

Meanwhile, there exists a high imbalance in the practice of LLR geographically and individually. Some leading surgeons have already successfully completed the anatomically accurate segmentectomy of all the Couinaud segments, which almost eliminated the absolute technical contraindications of LLR (Ishizawa et al. 2012). In most of the other hospitals, LLR remains to be a technically challenging surgery and the peripheral non-anatomic liver resections are more preferred to perform laparoscopically. LLR has not become a standardization operation, because the complications may be more difficult to control laparoscopically than the procedure itself. The relative contraindications of LLR are changed with the advances of surgeons' techniques. There is still a long way to achieve the standardization and promotion of LLR.

1.1 What is LAH?

Laparoscopic anatomical hepatectomy (LAH), instead of laparoscopic regular hepatectomy, according to our experience, stands for the laparoscopic regional resection of hepatic tumor or hepatic segment(s), based on the regional control of blood supply (Fig. 1.2), which is more technical complicated than open anatomical hepatectomy. Generally speaking, it means a surgical idea that we have to control the blood supply before resection of the tumor. For regular resection, LAH means effective inflow and outflow blood control before resection, and for irregular resection, it means effective feeding vessel control before resection.

LAH often requires more special techniques. To better expose the target region and critical anatomic structure of the liver, the patient position and trocar distribution should be arranged jointly and flexibly, which leads to a series of innovations such as trans-thoracic LAH (Hallet et al. 2015) and retroperitoneal LLR (Hu et al. 2011). Laparoscopic intraoperative ultrasonography is important for laparoscopic anatomical hepatectomy, especially for those less experienced surgeons, which is the last chance for a surgeon to confirm the intrahepatic structure before parenchyma dissection, including the location of the tumor and its spatial relationship with the major hepatic vessels, tumor-bearing portal pedicles, and landmark hepatic vein.

Anatomical hepatectomy (AH) has three technique characteristics: identification and transection of the portal pedicle, ischemic line-guided parenchyma dissection, and full exposure of related hepatic vein in the raw surface of the remnant liver. It is generally believed that REAL anatomical hepatectomy should possess these three features indispensably.

In our opinion, the three characteristics are not identical in terms of their importance. Identification and transection of the portal pedicle is the most fundamental step for anatomical hepatectomy, and usually constitutes the basis for the other two characteristics. Only if the portal pedicle is identified, the subsequent ischemic line could be revealed. The process of hepatic vein exposure is essential to the establishment of the cutting plane and parenchyma dissection. This is the most essential characteristic of anatomical hepatectomy.

With the understanding of the above, the concept of LAH could be expanded, with the main focus on the extent of resection, besides complete resection of the Couinaud segments and their combination. Wakabayashi brought up "laparoscopic limited anatomical resection" (Yoon et al. 2013), and used the limited anatomic sub-segmental resection to replace the central bisegmentectomy. The merits of LAH, such as less

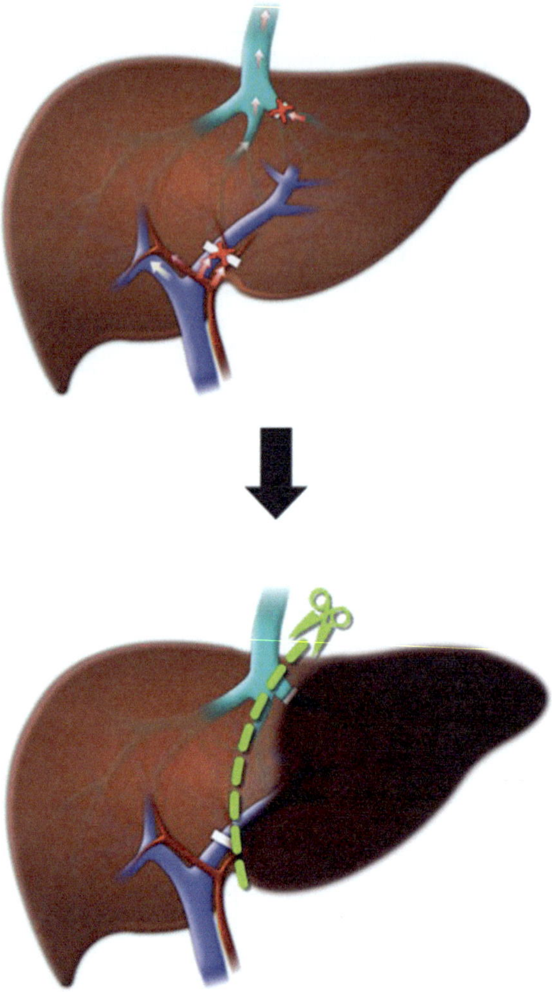

Fig. 1.2 The scheme of LAH

blood loss and clear cutting boundaries, have been inherited, while more normal liver parenchyma is preserved. Takahashi defined the subunit of Couinaud segments as a cone unit (Yamamoto et al. 2014). Each cone unit contains a single tertiary Glissonean branch and its territory parenchyma. Couinaud segments consist of three or four cone units. The idea deepened the understanding of the nature of LAH. Actually, exposure of the hepatic vein may be adopted by non-anatomic partial hepatectomy to guarantee the enough margin in LLR (Yoon et al. 2013).

According to our practical experience, to expose the full landmark hepatic vein is relatively demanding than identification of the portal pedicle and parenchyma dissection. If those surgeons with less experience recklessly dissect the parenchyma around the main hepatic vein, uncontrollable bleeding might be caused, which is more difficult to fix by the same surgeon laparoscopically. There essentially exist some compromises due to the level of current laparoscopic surgical practice. In fact, sufficient margin may play a more important role than exposure of the entire hepatic vein.

LAH should be a clinically feasible and flexible strategy, rather than to just find the boundaries and root according to the Couinaud liver segments. Laparoscopic anatomic hepatectomy is not equivalent to laparoscopic segmental resection or all sorts of their combination.

1.2 Why Choose LAH?

The role of LAH is built on its surgical and oncological values.

LAH could reduce intraoperative blood loss, decrease the incidence of postoperative biliary leak and other complications, minimize the loss of normal liver tissue, accelerate postoperative recovery, and provide the possibility of repeated liver resection. The parenchyma dissection by LAH is accompanied with a linear "vessel-less" plane. This decreases the injury possibility of the small branches of artery, portal vein, and bile duct. The irregular multidimensional transection plane of the non-anatomic liver resection could cause more unpredictable vessel injuries. Through a segment-based liver resection and its variants, we could preserve as much normal parenchyma as possible while ensure a enough surgical margin. The adequate margin is the key to prevent tumor recurrence, while enough liver preservation contributes a lot to postoperative recovery, especially for those with liver cirrhosis. LAH also causes less postoperative abdominal adhesions. Once tumor relapse occurs, repeated LAH could be performed. Most importantly, LAH can be used for tumors located at any region only if it is suitable for resection as discussed above, including those centrally located tumors (Yoon et al. 2013).

The patients of hepatocellular carcinoma (HCC) benefit markedly from anatomic hepatectomy oncologically. HCC has the pathologic features of spreading along the portal vein. Through complete resection of the liver section or segment with its portal pedicles, anatomic hepatectomy eliminates the potential intrahepatic metastasis of HCC as much as possible. The overall survival of HCC could be improved by anatomic hepatectomy (Hasegawa et al. 2005). It is well believed that the patients with metastatic tumor, such as colorectal liver metastasis (CRLM), may benefit less from anatomic hepatectomy than from HCC (Kokudo et al. 2001). However, there are some exceptions. For those CRLM's location is deep, LAH could prevent the parenchymal division from the positive margin. The tumor boundary could turn out to be fuzzy after the neoadjuvant chemotherapy. LAH could then become a more reasonable and reliable choice to guarantee sufficient surgical margin than non-anatomic hepatectomy.

LAH has the same inherited oncological value as the traditional open anatomic hepatectomy. Meanwhile, LAH also involves almost all the necessary techniques for laparoscopic non-anatomic hepatectomy, which in turn makes it become the fundamental technique for all laparoscopic liver resection. The standards of these basic techniques are relatively high and worthy of promoting.

1.3 Key Issues and Technique Details

1.3.1 Identification of Portal Pedicles and Root of Hepatic Vein

The main hepatic vessel control approaches, including the portal pedicles and root of hepatic vein, have been shown in Fig. 1.3. The simultaneous control of portal pedicles and hepatic vein, as the inflow and outflow vessels respectively, is the classic pattern of "bloodless" hepatectomy.

There are essentially three approaches for identification and transection of the portal pedicles: hilar access approach, Glissonean pedicle approach, and fissural approach (Yamamoto et al. 2014).

The hilar access approach means the dissection is in the sheath between the hepatoduodenal ligament and hilar plate. It is an extrahepatic approach without dissection of the liver parenchyma. With this approach, the secondary branches of the liver artery, portal vein, and bile duct could be dissected and controlled separately. The hepatic parenchyma could be often dissected and surgeon should try to control the tertiary branches of the hilus vessels at the same time. The hilar access approach is a delicate and demanding surgical procedure. Due to the common variations of hepatic artery (Figs. 1.4 and 1.5) and bile duct, the dissection in the fascia could be dangerous. The injuries to the hilus artery and portal vein might cause drastic consequences.

The hilar access approach was used mainly in the early stage of LAH. It has been considered to be time consuming and difficult to master. This technique may be more suitable for radical lymphadenectomy of the liver hilus rather than the liver resection itself.

The Glissonean pedicle approach can be achieved with or without parenchyma dissection. The extrahepatic approach (usually for hemihepatectomy and sectionectomy) is relatively easier than the intrahepatic approach (usually for segmentectomy), and thereby determines that the segmentectomy is more challenging than the major hepatectomy. Due to the essence of extra-fascial dissection, the Glissonean pedicle approach is much safer than the hilar access approach for less incidence of injury to the hilar vessels (Yamamoto et al. 2014).

The extrahepatic Glissonean pedicle approach is commonly used in the secondary branches near the hilus. The Glisson's capsule between the hilar plate and liver substance is incised, with the help of gentle opposite traction of the quadrant lobe and hepatoduodenal ligament. The confluence of secondary portal pedicles was then exposed and easy to manipulate. A common scenario is that the confluence of anterior and posterior portal pedicle is revealed at same time. After transection of one of the secondary portal pedicles, the relevant ischemic demarcation line becomes observable.

The intrahepatic Glissonean pedicle approach is usually used in the segmentectomy such as the segments 2, 4a, 5, 6, 7, and 8. When the portal pedicles of the segment are hard to control out of the liver substance, the parenchyma is dissected along an assumed boundary line to find the root of the portal pedicles. This line could be roughly determined with the help of the hepatic surface landmark or

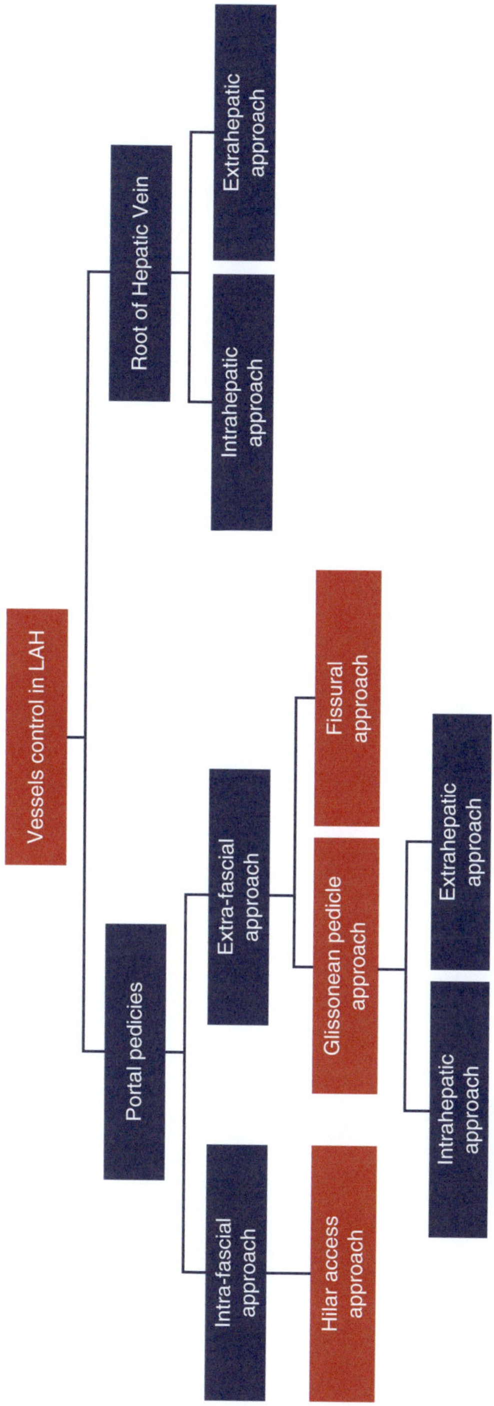

Fig. 1.3 Classification of main vessel control approaches of LAH

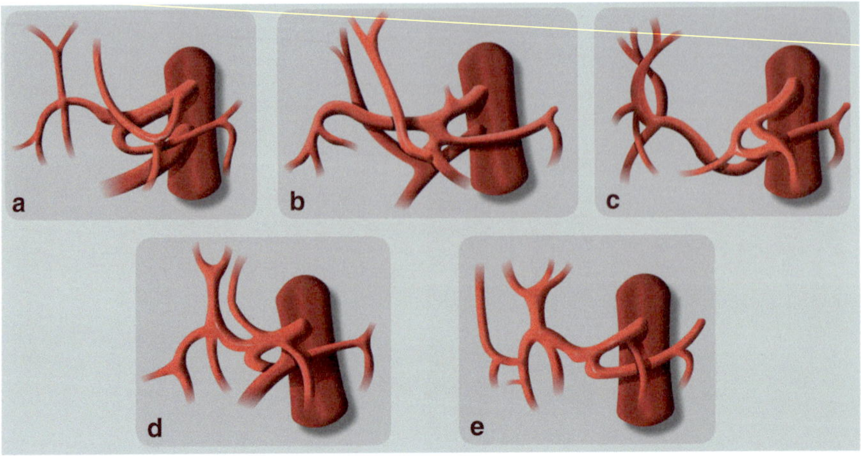

Fig. 1.4 Variations of extrahepatic arteries

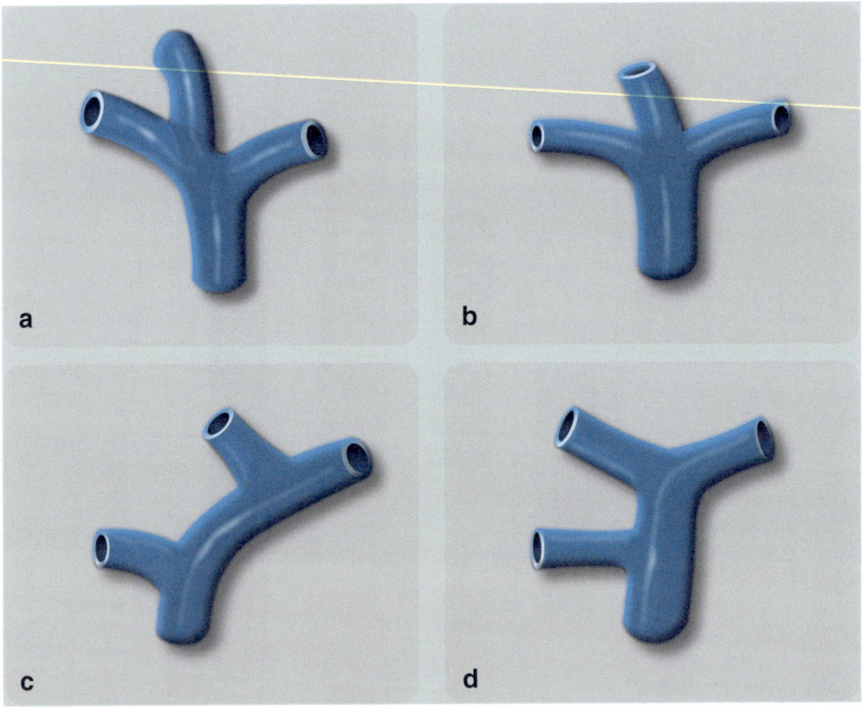

Fig. 1.5 Variations of extrahepatic portal veins

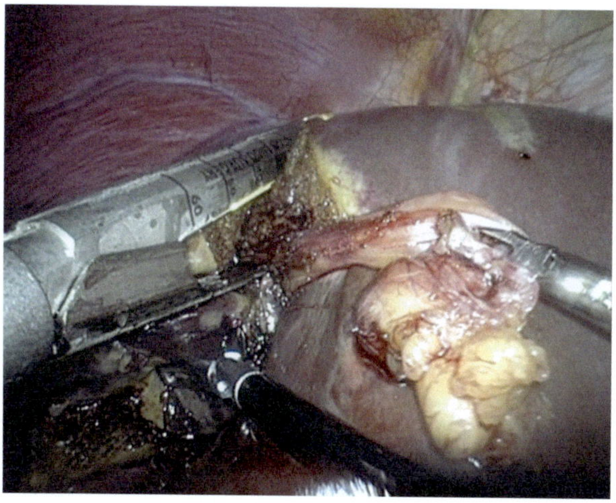

Fig. 1.6 Fissural approach

intraoperative ultrasonography. So the primary cutting line need not be too long. After transection of the pedicles, segmentectomy then could be finished along the relatively more accurate ischemic line.

Compared with the hilar access approach, the Glissonean pedicle approach is easier to handle and safer (Machado et al. 2011).

The fissural approach is mostly fit for the segmentectomy such as the segments 3 and 4b (Fig. 1.6). The umbilical fissure could be opened with or even without slight liver substance dissection, and the pedicles of segments 3 and 4b are then confirmed. The fissural approach is special transformation of the Glissonean pedicle approach.

There exists another way to handle the portal pedicles as in the laparoscopic left lateral sectionectomy (Chang et al. 2007). This procedure needs neither hilar incision or liver parenchyma dissection nor the navigation of ultrasound or dyeing. It simplifies dependence on the landmark of liver to achieve anatomic hepatectomy. With the limited indications and simple operations, this method is easy to promote. The details are shown in relevant chapter.

Identification of the root of hepatic vein could also be implemented in the intrahepatic and extrahepatic approach (Figs. 1.7 and 1.8). The extra approach is necessarily accompanied with a full liver mobilization. The intrahepatic approach involves ligation of the root of hepatic vein during the parenchyma dissection. The latter approach is believed to be faster and easier to operate (Toro et al. 2015).

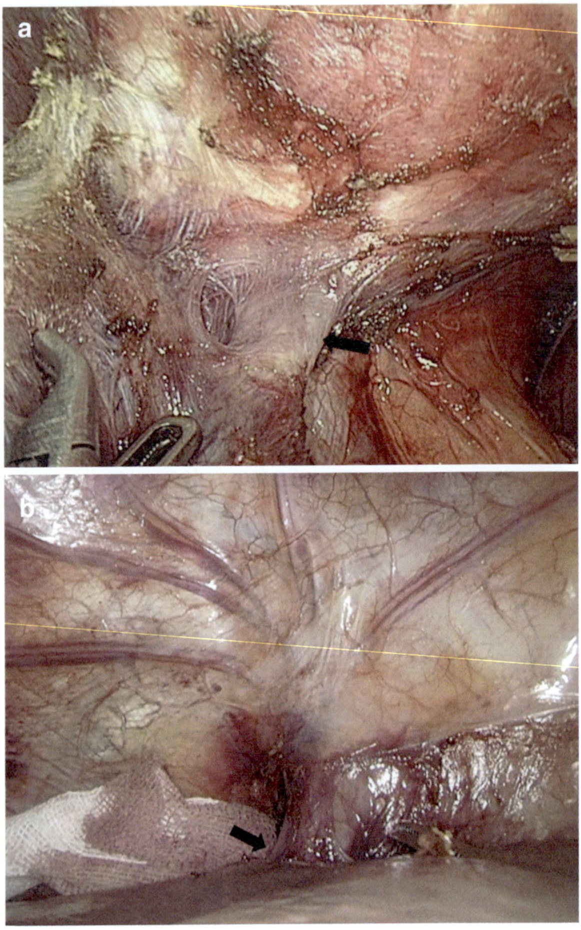

Fig. 1.7 Extrahepatic Approach of identification of the root of hepatic vein (**a**) Left hepatic vein (*arrow*) and (**b**) Right hepatic vein (*arrow*)

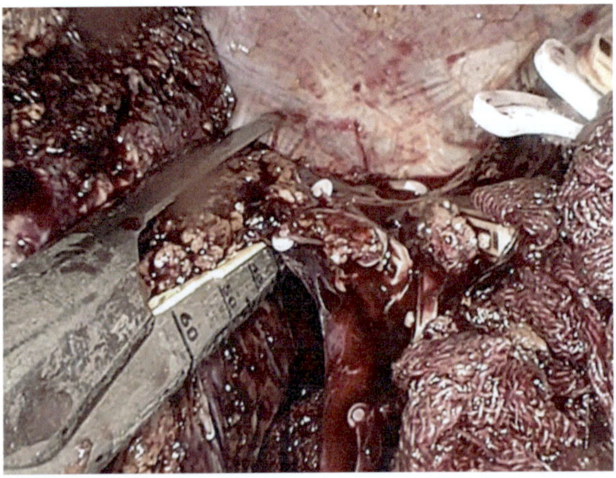

Fig. 1.8 Intrahepatic Approach of identification of the root of hepatic vein

1.3.2 Prevention of Bleeding and Hemostasis

Bleeding is still the most important issue limiting the improvement of laparoscopic liver resection (Shelat et al. 2015). The massive intraoperative blood loss along with later blood transfusion would greatly damage the patients' immune system, affect their postoperative recovery, and make tumors more likely to relapse. And it is also the most common reason for the conversion to open surgery (Abu Hilal et al. 2010). The prevention and control of bleeding during laparoscopic hepatectomy is achieved by a number of integrated measures.

Measures to prevent bleeding is more important than those to stop bleeding (Fig. 1.9). LAH itself is a fundamental method to prevent bleeding through ensuring a "bloodless" cutting plane and controlling the inflow and outflow vessels as discussed above. Other favorable measures include carbon dioxide pneumoperitoneum, low central venous pressure and airway pressure. Careful examination and meticulous hemostasis should be consistently carried out throughout the whole operation.

In face of bleeding, surgical members may have many options including bipolar coagulation, vessel sealing devices, titanium clips, vascular locks, staplers, and suture. The vessel-dependent indications should be clear for different measures (Wakabayashi et al. 2015). Laparoscopic suture skill is the key to ensure the safety of LAH. Without it, the complicated laparoscopic surgery would be a dangerous speculation (Shelat et al. 2015).

When no progress is made in a certain period, conversion should be considered. Conversion to open surgery should not be regarded as complication, but reasonable surgical decision (Dagher et al. 2009).

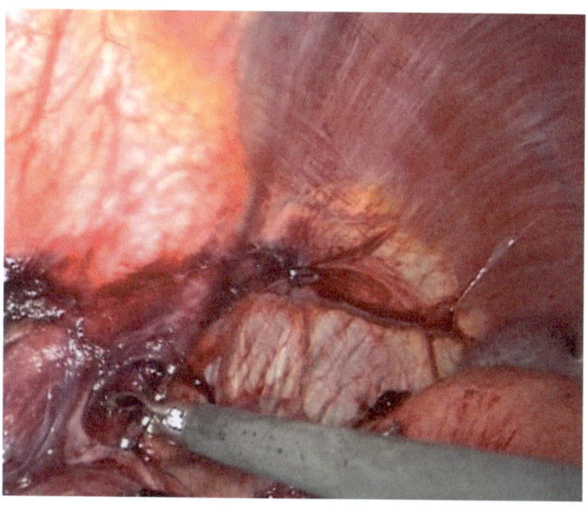

Fig. 1.9 Ligation of left inferior phrenic vein before dissecting left hepatic vein

1.3.3 Parenchymal Dissection and Exposure of Hepatic Vein

The process of liver parenchymal dissection involves formation of the liver cutting plane and exposure of the hepatic vein in LAH. The key is to find the right boundary between the adjacent territories of the portal pedicels. The target specimen should contain the tumor completely and the cancer-free liver parenchyma should be reserved as much as possible.

Many energy devices and mechanical staples could be used in laparoscopic liver parenchymal transection. The employed techniques are usually individualized from different surgeons. Up until now, there is no clear evidence that a certain device or technique is more advantageous (Dagher et al. 2009). It is vital that surgeons have a reliable insight into the merits and defects of devices and techniques available to perform safe and efficient LAH. The flexible combination of various methods and devices may be the best solution under the present conditions. The basic liver surgery techniques are still the cornerstone of LAH, including delicate dissection, enough exposure of the surgical field, and vascular suture skills (Wakabayashi et al. 2015).

M. A. Machado divided the transection plane of pure laparoscopic right hemihepatectomy into three continuous parts: anterior, middle, and posterior parts (Machado et al. 2011) (Fig. 1.10).

The three parts involve different containing vessels inside and subsequent transection methods. There is no main vessel in the anterior part. It can be divided by ultrasonic scalpel along the ischemic line (Fig. 1.11). There exist hepatic short veins in the posterior part. A staple should be used to transect this part as a whole (Fig. 1.12). There are the right secondary main portal pedicles, the root of the RHV and the considerable branches of the MHV in the middle part (Fig. 1.13). This part should be transected with staples after the anterior and posterior parts. Such division and sequence have brought LAH more safe and clear guidance (Machado et al. 2011).

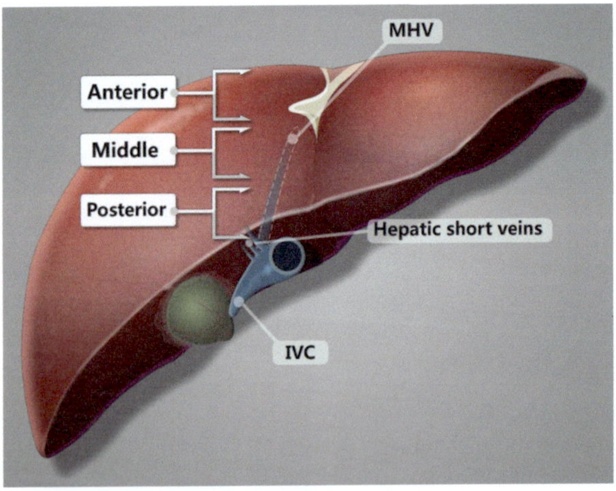

Fig. 1.10 Three parts of the transection plane of laparoscopic right hemihepatectomy

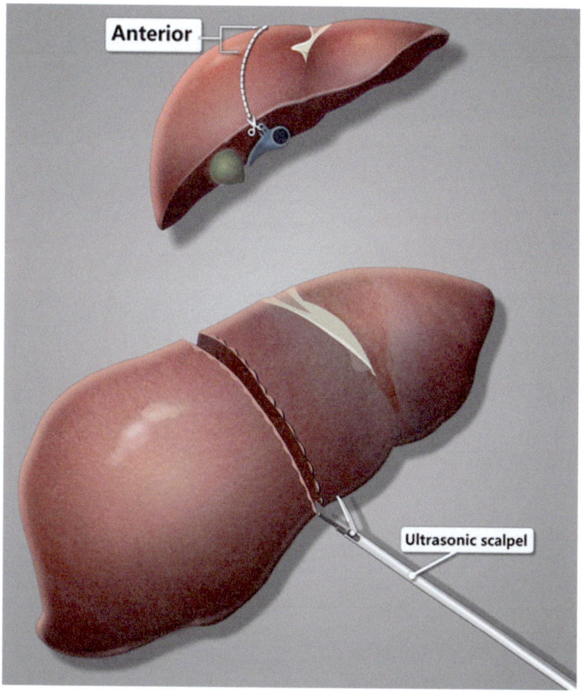

Fig. 1.11 Transection of the anterior part

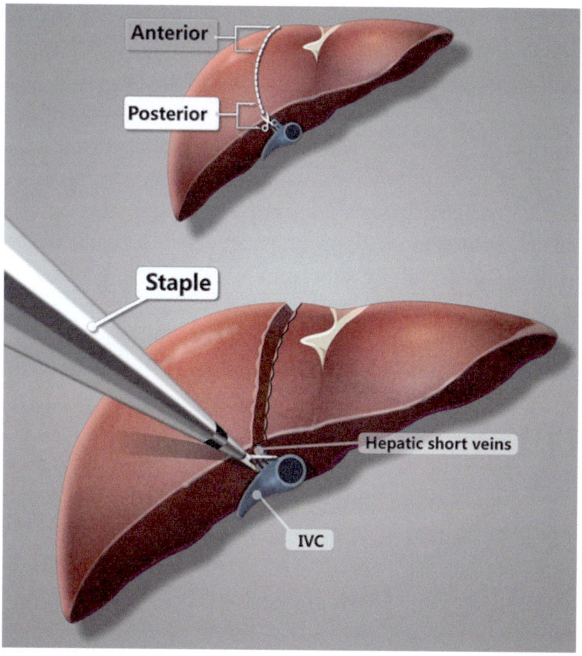

Fig. 1.12 Transection of the posterior part

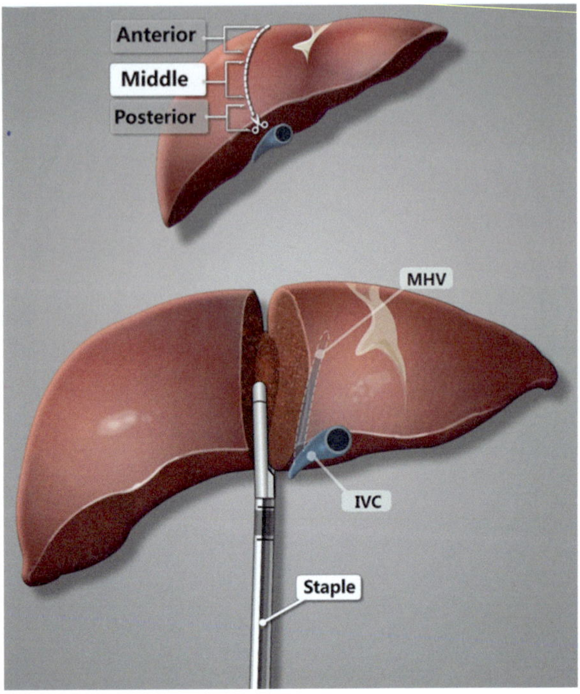

Fig. 1.13 Transection of the middle part

The Couinaud segments are surrounded by the hepatic veins. The real anatomic hepatectomy unavoidably involves exposure of the major hepatic veins on the cutting plane. The complete exposure of intrahepatic hepatic veins is the essence of hepatectomy. This also applies to LAH (Ishizawa et al. 2012).

Before start, all measures for prevention and control of bleeding should be adopted as mentioned above in case of massive bleeding. The clamp crushing technique is still the basic skill to expose the hepatic veins as in open liver resection. The tips of laparoscopic instruments are used to get rid of the hepatic substance adhering to the venous wall by short reciprocated scrape (Ishizawa et al. 2012). The direction of movement should be from the root to the peripheral, considering the inverted tree-shape of hepatic vein (Honda et al. 2014).

1.3.4 Intraoperative Navigation

Intraoperative navigation provides functions of locating the liver tumor and its relationship with intrahepatic vessel structures and guiding the consequent hepatectomy. The ultrasonography is the most important means of intraoperative navigation. The target portal pedicles could be found by intraoperative ultrasonography. And then the ischemic or discoloration line could be demonstrated by transection

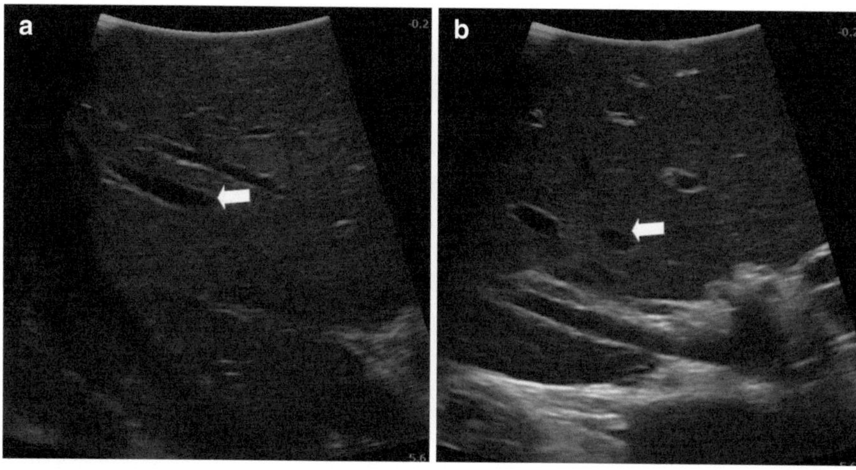

Fig. 1.14 The routine examination order of laparoscopic intraoperative ultrasonography (**a**) Longitudinal inspection; (**b**) Horizontal inspection

or dyeing. In recent researches, the fluorescein staining technique and augmented reality technique have been used for the same purpose (Hallet et al. 2015).

The laparoscopic intraoperative ultrasonography is the key of LAH. Unlike the flexibility in the open surgery, it is usually relatively fixed on the root of the detection probe by trocar. A routine examination order is necessary to avoid any missed diagnosis.

There are two basic inspection dimensionalities in laparoscopic intraoperative ultrasonography: longitudinal and horizontal (Fig. 1.14). The longitudinal inspection is to move the ultrasound probe from the left to the right on the hepatic diaphragmatic surface. The long axis section of the left hepatic vein, middle hepatic vein, retrohepatic inferior vena cava, and right hepatic vein will be shown on the monitor in turn. The horizontal inspection is to move the ultrasound probe from the top to the liver edge on the hepatic diaphragmatic surface. When the divisions of the superior and inferior branches of the secondary portal vein are found, the borders between 4a and 4b, 5 and 8, 6 and 7 are then identified. The position of the laparoscopic ultrasonography trocar should be carefully chosen in order to make the whole liver available (Ishizawa et al. 2012).

Fluorescence imaging is also very useful in the intraoperative guidance of LLR, which has been widely used since the late 2000s (Ishizawa et al. 2009). Based on the dynamic ICG imaging, we developed a novel and feasible intraoperative guiding method, which is named as tri-phase quadri-sectional imaging (TPQSI), which can identify four anatomic sections during LLR (Fig. 1.15), including tumor, paraneoplastic area, ischemic area, and remnant area. Briefly, before surgery, ICG dye was injected intravenously, and during the operation, tumor and paraneoplastic area on the surface of liver would emit a pseudocolor-green light on the fusion images mode

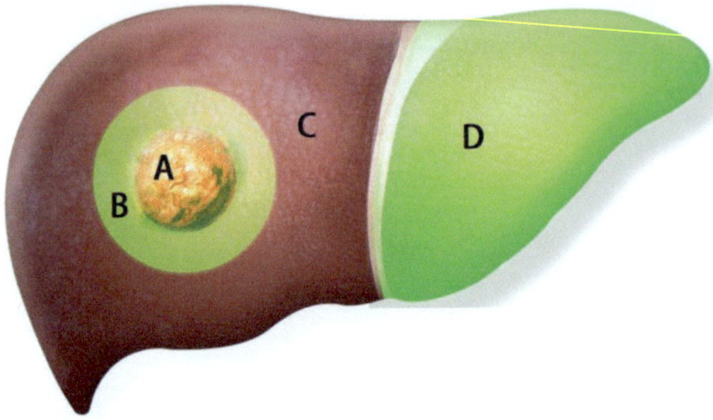

Fig. 1.15 The four anatomic sections demonstrated using tri-phase quadri-sectional imaging. (**a**) tumor; (**b**) paraneoplastic area; (**c**) ischemic area; (**d**) remnant area

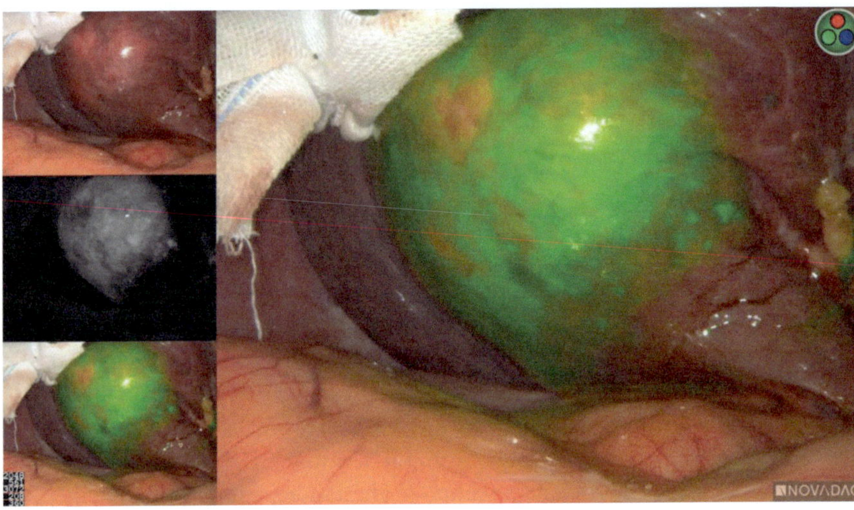

Fig. 1.16 A 6-cm tumor and the paraneoplastic area in segment 5 and 8 were identified by fusion IGFI

(Fig. 1.16) (sometimes there is not a clear line between these two areas). A significant benefit is that IGFI could identify tiny subcapsular hepatic malignancies not detected by visual inspection (Kudo et al. 2014) or conventional imaging modalities (Terasawa et al. 2017), although deep-located tumors should be diagnosed by laparoscopic intraoperative ultrasonography. After controlling the inflow of right liver, ICG was intravenously injected, and the ischemic line on the liver surface would appear, which divides the liver into two areas, the ischemic area and the remnant area (Fig. 1.17). According to the staining boundaries, LAH could be performed under a real-time navigation (Fig. 1.18).

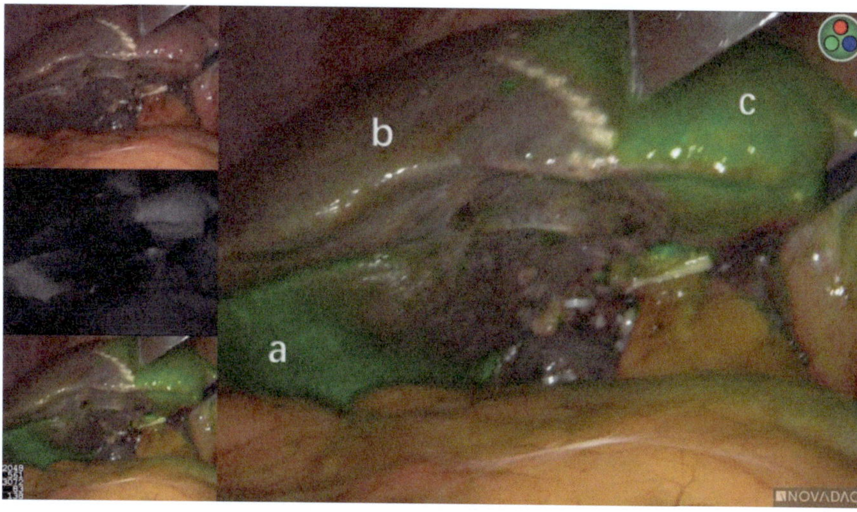

Fig. 1.17 TPQSI after blood control: (**a**) tumor and paraneoplastic area; (**b**) unstaining section; (**c**) remnant-staining section

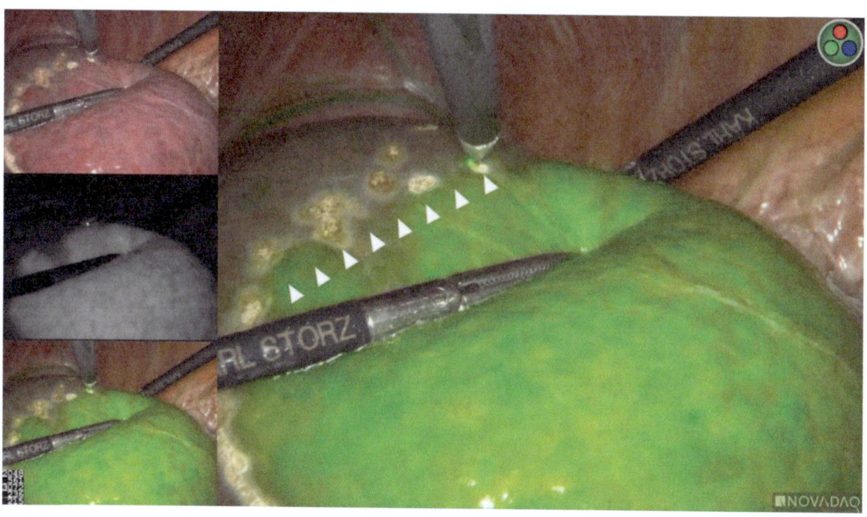

Fig. 1.18 TPQSI after blood control: transection line based on the boundaries between section b and c

With the help of laparoscopic intraoperative ultrasonography and TPQSI, the accuracy of LAH is enhanced, and more tumor-free parenchyma is preserved while the adequate surgical margin is also secured.

References

Abu Hilal M, et al. Bleeding and hemostasis in laparoscopic liver surgery. Surg Endosc. 2010;24(3):572–7.

Chang S, et al. Laparoscopy as a routine approach for left lateral sectionectomy. Br J Surg. 2007;94(1):58–63.

Dagher I, et al. Laparoscopic major hepatectomy: an evolution in standard of care. Ann Surg. 2009;250(5):856–60.

Hallet J, et al. Trans-thoracic minimally invasive liver resection guided by augmented reality. J Am Coll Surg. 2015;220(5):e55–60.

Hasegawa K, et al. Prognostic impact of anatomic resection for hepatocellular carcinoma. Ann Surg. 2005;242(2):252–9.

Honda G, et al. Totally laparoscopic anatomical hepatectomy exposing the major hepatic veins from the root side: a case of the right anterior sectorectomy (with video). J Gastrointest Surg. 2014;18(7):1379–80.

Hu M, et al. Retroperitoneal laparoscopic hepatectomy: a novel approach. Surg Laparosc Endosc Percutan Tech. 2011;21(5):e245–8.

Ishizawa T, et al. Real-time identification of liver cancers by using indocyanine green fluorescent imaging. Cancer. 2009;115(11):2491–504.

Ishizawa T, et al. Laparoscopic segmentectomy of the liver: from segment I to VIII. Ann Surg. 2012;256(6):959–64.

Kokudo N, et al. Anatomical major resection versus nonanatomical limited resection for liver metastases from colorectal carcinoma. Am J Surg. 2001;181(2):153–9.

Kudo H, et al. Visualization of subcapsular hepatic malignancy by indocyanine-green fluorescence imaging during laparoscopic hepatectomy. Surg Endosc. 2014;28(8):2504–8.

Machado MA, Surjan RC, Makdissi FF. Video: intrahepatic Glissonian approach for pure laparoscopic right hemihepatectomy. Surg Endosc. 2011;25(12):3930–3.

Shelat VG, et al. Pure laparoscopic liver resection for large malignant tumors: does size matter? Ann Surg Oncol. 2015;22(4):1288–93.

Terasawa M, et al. Applications of fusion-fluorescence imaging using indocyanine green in laparoscopic hepatectomy. Surg Endosc. 2017. https://doi.org/10.1007/s00464-017-5576-z.

Toro JP, et al. Detecting performance variance in complex surgical procedures: analysis of a stepwise technique for laparoscopic right hepatectomy. Am J Surg. 2015;209(2):418–23.

Wakabayashi G, et al. Recommendations for laparoscopic liver resection: a report from the second international consensus conference held in Morioka. Ann Surg. 2015;261(4):619–29.

Yamamoto M, et al. Tips for anatomical hepatectomy for hepatocellular carcinoma by the Glissonean pedicle approach (with videos). J Hepatobiliary Pancreat Sci. 2014;21(8):E53–6.

Yoon YS, et al. Laparoscopic liver resection for centrally located tumors close to the hilum, major hepatic veins, or inferior vena cava. Surgery. 2013;153(4):502–9.

Patient Positioning and Ports Placement

2

Abstract

Patient Positioning and Ports Placement are important to laparoscopic liver resection. Ports placement for this procedure requires careful preoperative planning based on the anatomic location of the hepatic lesion. We suggest three different positions according to the lesion site.

Patient Positioning and Ports Placement are important to laparoscopic liver resection. Ports placement for this procedure requires careful preoperative planning based on the anatomic location of the hepatic lesion. We suggest three different positions according to the lesion site.

2.1 Patient Position

2.1.1 The First Position: Reverse Trendelenburg Position

The patient is placed in supine position with a 20-degree reverse-Trendelenburg adjustment, which is suitable for the majority of laparoscopic liver surgery (Fig. 2.1).

Methods: The surgeon stands on the opposite side of the lesion (e.g., if lesion in the left lateral lobe, the surgeon stands on the right side of the patient). The first assistant stands on the other side of the patient. This position is appropriate for the majority of laparoscopic liver surgery, such as local hepatectomy, left lateral lobectomy, left hemihepatectomy, etc.

2.1.2 The Second Position: Lithotomy Position

Methods: The patient is placed in the supine position, with lower limbs apart (Figs. 2.2 and 2.3), the surgeon stands between the legs with one assistant on each side. We use this position in single-port laparoscopic surgery.

R. Liu, *Laparoscopic Liver Resection*,
https://doi.org/10.1007/978-94-017-9735-1_2

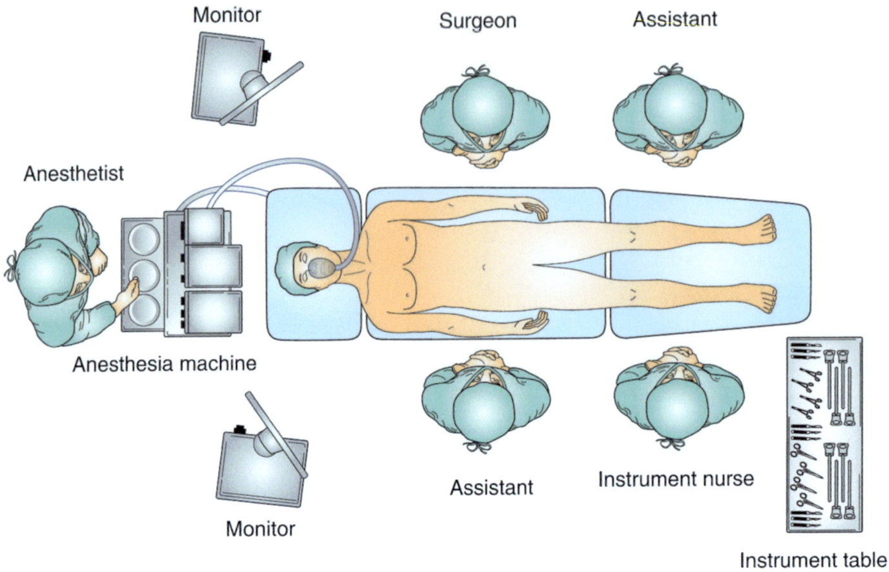

Fig. 2.1 Operating room setup of reverse Trendelenburg position

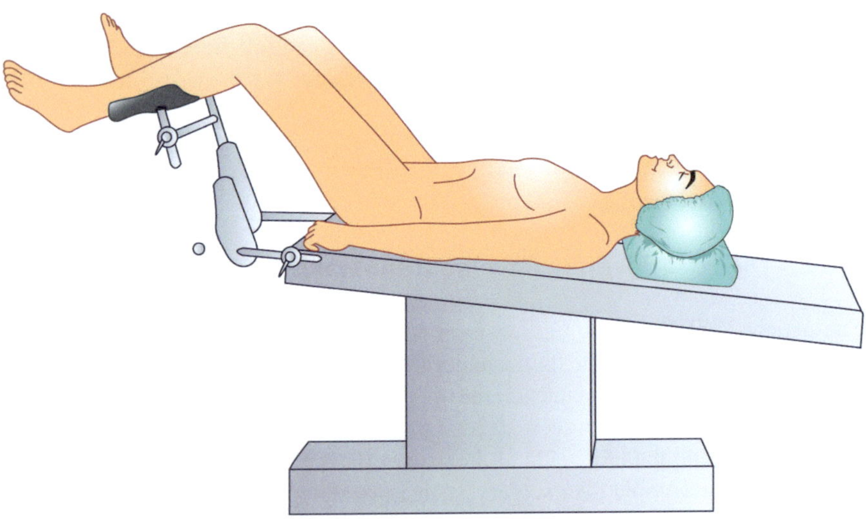

Fig. 2.2 The side view of lithotomy position

2.1.3 The Third Position: Left Lateral Decubitus Position

The left lateral decubitus position with a steep reverse Trendelenburg position is ideal for lesions in the right lobe—particularly those requiring mobilization of the right lobe to gain access to the posterior surface (Fig. 2.4).

Fig. 2.3 The front view of lithotomy position

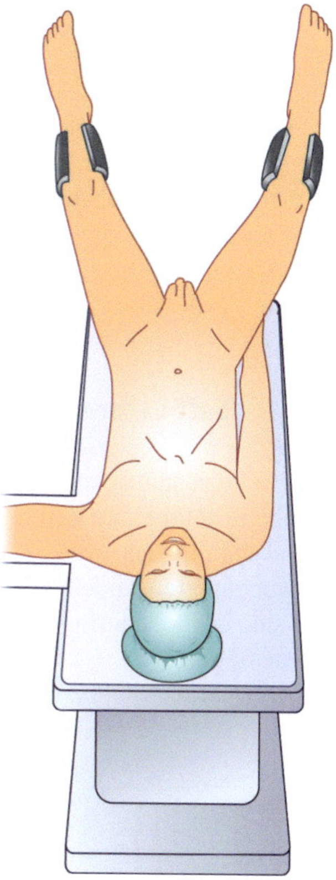

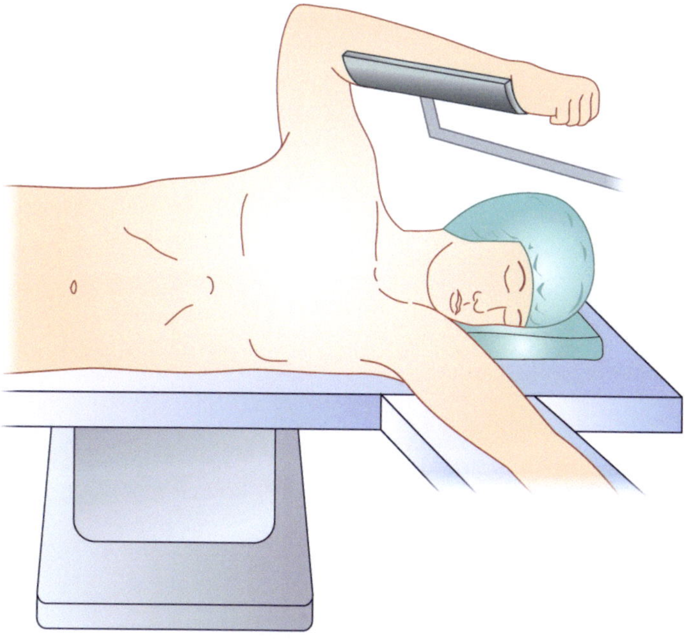

Fig. 2.4 The side view of left lateral decubitus position

2.2 Principle of Trocar Positioning

Positioning of port sites is different according to the tumor site. When the patient is placed in position, pneumoperitoneum is achieved through a Veress needle under the umbilicus to insufflate the peritoneal cavity to 14 mmHg. A first 10-mm trocar is then placed under the umbilicus for laparoscope. The other two 12-mm trocars are located in the upper abdomen, according to the location of the tumor. Besides the two 12-mm trocars, a 5-mm trocar is then placed assisting in organ exposure, traction, and suction.

2.2.1 Left Lateral Lobectomy and Left Hemihepatectomy

The surgeon stands on the right side of the patient, and the first main operating port is located on the junction between the right midclavicular line and 4 cm below the costal margin. The second main operating port position is located on the junction between the left midclavicular line and a little bit below the costal margin. On the left side of the anterior axillary line to establish assistant operation hole for 5 mm trocar (Fig. 2.5).

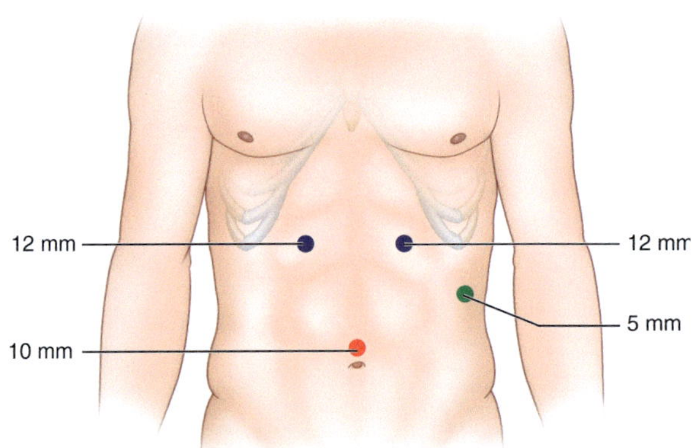

Fig. 2.5 Port position for left lateral lobectomy and left hemihepatectomy

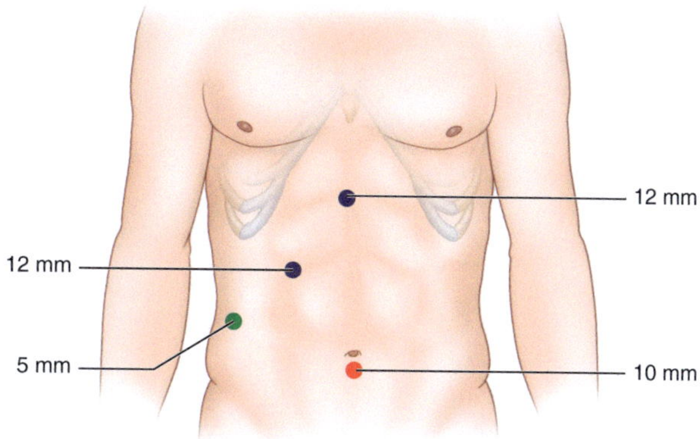

Fig. 2.6 Port position for right posterior lobectomy

2.2.2 Right Posterior Lobectomy

The surgeon stands on the left side of the patient, and the first main operating port is located on the junction between the right midclavicular line and 4 cm below the costal margin. The second main operating port position is located below xiphoid bone. On the right anterior axillary line and 4 cm above the level of umbilicus, a 5 mm trocar is then introduced to establish an assistant operating port (Fig. 2.6).

2.2.3 Right Hemihepatectomy

The surgeon stands on the left side of the patient, and the first main operating port is located on the junction between the right midclavicular line and 4 cm below the costal margin. The second main operating port is located on the junction between the left midclavicular line and a little bit below the costal margin. On the right anterior axillary line and 4 cm above the level of umbilicus, a 5 mm trocar is introduced to establish an assistant operating port (Fig. 2.7).

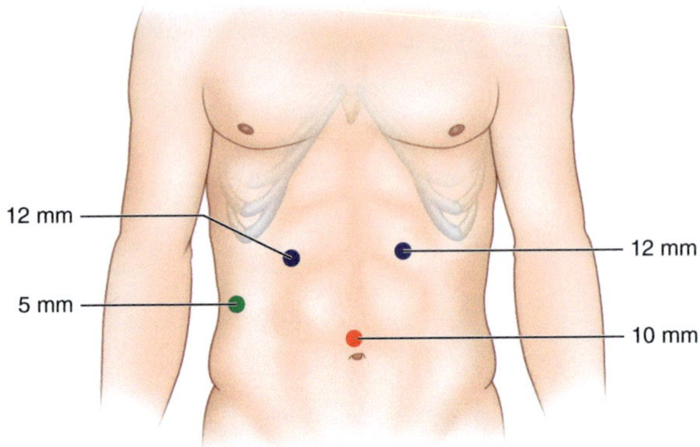

Fig. 2.7 Port position for right hemihepatectomy

3 Preoperative Preparation and Anesthesia for Laparoscopic Liver Resection

Abstract
It is very important to do adequate preparation before surgery for laparoscopic liver resection. Strict case selection and surgical instrument preparation play important roles in the preparation. In this chapter, we focus on the preparation of patients and surgical instruments, and give a brief introduction to the selection of anesthesia.

It is very important to do adequate preparation before surgery for laparoscopic liver resection. Strict case selection and surgical instrument preparation play important roles in the preparation. In this chapter, we focus on the preparation of patients and surgical instruments, and give a brief introduction to the selection of anesthesia.

3.1 Preoperative Evaluation of Patients

After admission, the patient who will receive laparoscopic liver resection should be evaluated for general state and nutritional status, and measures should be taken to correct the anemia, low serum albumin, and water electrolyte imbalance and to improve the nutritional status and liver function. Also, according to the imaging examination, the location, size, nature, etc. of the liver lesion should be seriously assessed to confirm indications for surgery. At the same time, a comprehensive assessment of heart, liver, lung, and other organs function will contribute to recognize contraindications of surgery.

3.1.1 Imaging Examination

3.1.1.1 Ultrasonography

Ultrasonography is a procedure used for liver tumor screening. The results of ultrasound examination are subjective and relevant to the expertise of the operator and technical limitations, thus ultrasonography can't be used to determine the surgical approaches.

R. Liu, *Laparoscopic Liver Resection*,
https://doi.org/10.1007/978-94-017-9735-1_3

Intraoperative ultrasound is necessary to laparoscopic liver surgery, especially in the local resection of liver tumors.

3.1.1.2 CT

CT can clearly show the density difference between liver lesions and the liver parenchyma. It also shows the blood supply of lesions and its internal structure. Cross-section reconstruction and three-dimensional reconstruction can be achieved by CT scan. Preoperative CT examination of liver disease is more accurate than ultrasonography.

3.1.1.3 MRI

The resolution of MRI is higher than CT, and there are a variety of imaging sequences. Besides, MRI has no radioactive damage and its contrast agent has less side effects. For liver cancer, especially small hepatocellular carcinoma (less than 2 cm), detection ability of MRI is better than that of CT. MRI is recommended as a routine use for liver tumor diagnosis.

3.1.1.4 PET-CT

PET-CT has obvious advantages in the identification of the nature of the tumor with the fluorine-18-FDG accumulating in the tissues of malignant tumor cells. PET-CT has an obvious advantage in the detection of extrahepatic lesions, which is beneficial for comprehensive preoperative staging of patients with malignant liver tumors. Due to the high cost, PET-CT is not used as the routine examination.

3.1.2 Systemic Organ Function Evaluation

3.1.2.1 Cardiac Function

Before laparoscopic liver resection, combine the patient's history and examination results (electrocardiogram and Doppler echocardiography, 24 h dynamic electrocardiogram, coronary angiography) to clarify whether there is surgical contraindication.

3.1.2.2 Respiratory Function

Pleural effusion, atelectasis, and pulmonary infection are common complications after liver resection. Due to a long time of pneumoperitoneum during surgery, laparoscopic surgery has more significant side effect on respiratory and circulation compared with open surgery, so the risk of respiratory system complication will be significantly increased in the patients with respiratory disease. According to the patients' blood gas analysis, pulmonary function examination results, objective evaluation of the respiratory system will be achieved. Respiratory function is also very difficult to greatly improve in a short period of time, therefore patients with respiratory system diseases should be carefully choose to undergo laparoscopic surgery.

3.1.2.3 Renal Function

Patients with liver cancer, especially hepatocellular carcinoma usually accompanied with chronic viral hepatitis and chronic liver damage, are prone to suffer postoperative ascites and even hepatorenal syndrome, etc. For patients with mild renal dysfunction, the electrolyte and acid–base balance disorder, low protein, etc. should be corrected appropriately before the operation. Meanwhile, for patients with liver cirrhosis, the perioperative infusion should be moderate, and it's beneficial to encourage patients to eat, so as to avoid fluid retention and renal insufficiency.

3.1.2.4 Liver Function

Under normal circumstances, the remnant liver after resection of 70–75% liver tissue could still maintain the normal physiological function of the liver. However, most of our patients with hepatocellular carcinoma (HCC) have chronic viral hepatitis, and in such patients, liver function is damaged to various degrees. After hepatic resection these patients are prone to postoperative liver function incomplete and even liver failure. Therefore, it is very important to assess the prognosis of patients with liver function and liver reserve function before liver resection. There are many methods to evaluate liver function, but there is no single method that can accurately and comprehensively reflect the severity of liver disease. The most basic method of preoperative liver function evaluation is the Child Turcotte Pugh (CTP) score of liver function which mainly includes five indicators (albumin, ascites, hepatic encephalopathy, bilirubin, and prothrombin time). According to the severity of the disease, each of the 5 indexes is counted as 1, 2, or 3, and the total score of 5 indexes can be divided into three grades: 5–6 points for Grade A, 7–9 points for grade B, and 10–15 points for C-class. It is generally believed that the patients with grade C in CTP score can hardly tolerate liver resection, and the mortality rate after liver resection of patients with grade B is significantly higher than that of the patients with Grade A. CTP score has the advantages of simple, practical, and economical. But the shortcomings of CTP score are also very obvious, for instance, no proper weight are taken into account among all these indicators, so it is hard to grade the ascites and hepatic encephalopathy. Indocyanine green clearance (IGG) is a synthetic, non-toxic, photosensitive dye in deep blue color. Due to its metabolic characteristics, the ICG excretion test is considered to be sensitive to the liver reserve function and is widely used in the field of liver resection. Combined application of CTP classification and the ICG excretive test may achieve a comprehensive and accurate assessment of liver function.

3.1.2.5 Patients with Psychological Expectations

All patients undergoing laparoscopic liver resection need to be prepared for conversion to open surgery. The possibility and necessity of conversion should be explained to patients and their families before operation.

3.2 Anesthesia in Laparoscopic Liver Resection

1. Before surgery, anesthesiologist should understand patient's medical history, evaluate patient's general state and the functions of important organs, so as to make sure there is no anesthetic contraindications. The anesthesiologist should also communicate with the surgeon to know operative strategy and what emergency may happen during the surgery.
2. Choice of anesthesia: Laparoscopic liver resection is generally adopted by general anesthesia under endotracheal intubation. Laparoscopic and endoscopic surgery experts suggested general anesthesia combined with epidural anesthesia in laparoscopic liver surgery, because epidural anesthesia can block afferent stimulation of injury during the operation and reduce the degree of stress response. For patients who have general anesthesia combined with epidural anesthesia and may get stable respiration and circulation during surgery, their postoperative recovery time and recovery quality is superior to that of patients with only general anesthesia. But if the patient is accompanied with cirrhosis and coagulation dysfunction, epidural puncture is likely to cause epidural hematoma. Anesthesia doctors should carefully select anesthesia method according to the specific circumstances of patients. General anesthesia can be induced by the standard drug, but after liver resection, the residual liver's ability to clear the anesthesia drug will be inhibited, so anesthesiologist should pay attention to the interaction between anesthetics and liver.
3. It's routine monitoring vital signs such as ECG, SpO2, and other indexes including urine volume, body temperature, blood glucose, electrolyte, blood coagulation function, and blood gas analysis. If the monitoring process is relatively complex, it is best to use invasive approach. For laparoscopic liver resection surgery, anesthesiologist not only deal with intraoperative bleeding problems during open hepatectomy, but also need to pay attention to persistent CO_2 pneumoperitoneum. To reduce the side effect of pneumoperitoneum on the body is crucial for anesthesiologist during the operation. In pneumoperitoneum state, the pathophysiological changes including large amount of CO_2 absorbed by peritoneal, an increase in intra-abdominal pressure, diaphragmatic elevation, increased airway pressure, and reduced lung capacity, could lead to pulmonary ventilation perfusion imbalance, hypercapnia, and acidosis. Therefore, monitoring of $PaCO_2$ is significant.

4 Laparoscopic Liver Cysts Fenestration

Abstract

Surgical treatments for liver cysts include: fenestration, liver resection with fenestration, regular hepatectomy, liver transplantation, and so on. Comparing with laparotomy, laparoscopic surgery has some advantages, including minimal invasiveness, short surgery time, quick recovery, simple operation, which may be the reason why laparoscopic fenestration has become the most popular method for liver cysts treatment. However, attention should be paid that for hepatic cystadenoma, hepatic cystadenocarcinoma, and hepatic cystic echinococcosis, open hepatectomy is still the optimal treatment.

Surgical treatments for liver cysts include: fenestration, liver resection with fenestration, regular hepatectomy, liver transplantation, and so on. Comparing with laparotomy, laparoscopic surgery has some advantages, including minimal invasiveness, short surgery time, quick recovery, simple operation, which may be the reason why laparoscopic fenestration has become the most popular method for liver cysts treatment. However, attention should be paid that for hepatic cystadenoma, hepatic cystadenocarcinoma, and hepatic cystic echinococcosis, open hepatectomy is still the optimal treatment.

4.1 Indications and Contraindications

4.1.1 Indications

1. Symptomatic liver cyst (non-parasitic and non-malignant)
2. Located on the surface of the liver
3. No communication with bile ducts
4. Single or multiple liver cysts
5. Sudden enlargement in cyst's volume (>10 cm)

R. Liu, *Laparoscopic Liver Resection*,
https://doi.org/10.1007/978-94-017-9735-1_4

4.1.2 Contraindication

1. Communication with bile ducts
2. Liver cystadenoma or cystadenocarcinoma
3. Parasitic liver cysts
4. Bacterial liver abscess
5. Suspected malignant tumors

4.2 Procedure

1. *Position and trocars' locations*: The patient is placed in supine position with surgeons between the patient's legs. A 10 mm trocar is placed via an infra-umbilical incision. Then a pressure-controlled CO_2 pneumoperitoneum is maintained at 12–14 mmHg, with end-tidal CO_2 concentration monitored continuously. Through this port, a 30° laparoscope is introduced to detect abdominal viscera overall and make sure the lesion's location. Then, according to its location, two additional trocars are inserted at suitable sites. When the surgeon puncturing abdominal wall, ensure trocar's sharp point under your sight in case of abdominal or retroperitoneal organs injury.
2. *Laparoscopy and intervention*: A laparoscope is introduced to have a further determination of lesions' site, number, interface relations between liver and cysts. When the lesion is confirmed as simple liver cyst, we usually use a monopolar electrocoagulation or ultrasonic dissector to incise a 5 mm hole on the cyst wall. Then a sucker is punctured to aspirate intra-cystic fluid out (Fig. 4.1). When necessary, it is recommended to have a laparoscopic fluid collection with needle to determine fluid quality (bile, mucus) firstly. If the lesion is suspected as a non-simple cyst preoperatively, the intra-cystic fluid should be examined pathologically, bacteriologically, biochemically.
3. *Cysts fenestration*: Deroofing is performed by monopolar electrocoagulation forceps or ultrasonic dissector or by Ligasure (Fig. 4.2). A sucker is positioned to aspirate the residual liquid. After above procedures, a cautious observation of

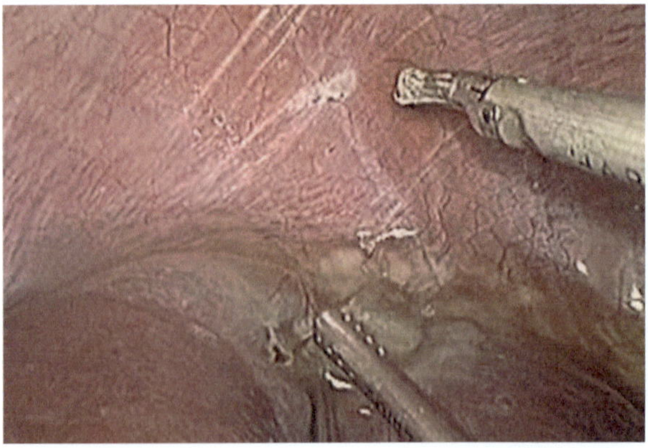

Fig. 4.1 Incise the cyst using ultrasounic scalpel and aspirate intra-cystic fluid out

the cyst wall is needed. If there are relatively thick vessels on the wall, it's recommended to occlude proximal bile ducts of these vessels so as to avoid bile leak (Fig. 4.3). The purpose of the surgery is sufficient fenestration, so that liver resection along the lesion's line is not essential (Fig. 4.4). For polycystic liver

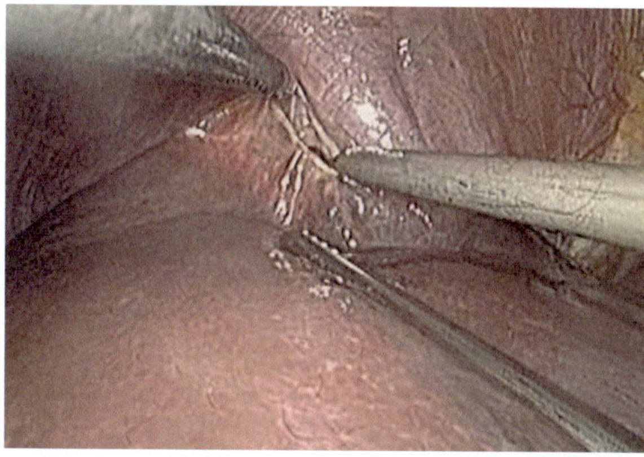

Fig. 4.2 Deroof the cyst and resect the cystic wall

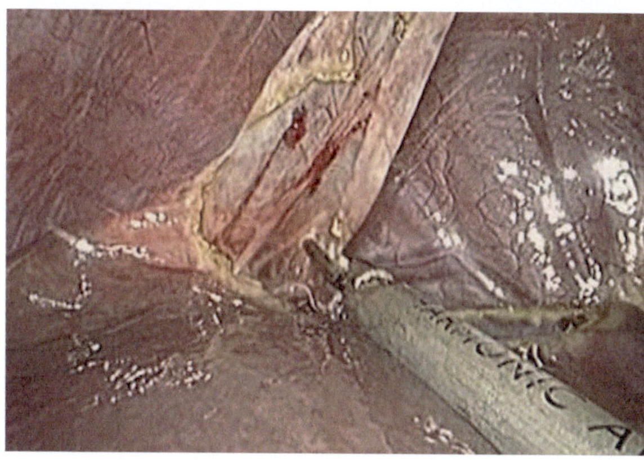

Fig. 4.3 Resect the whole cystic wall

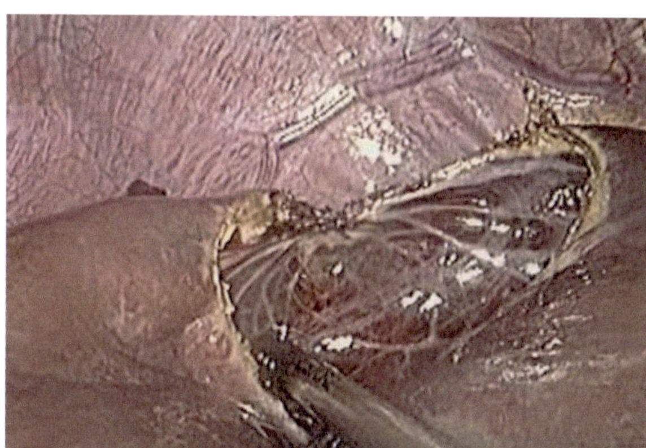

Fig. 4.4 After the deroofing, the cystic cavity shows multiple fibrous septa

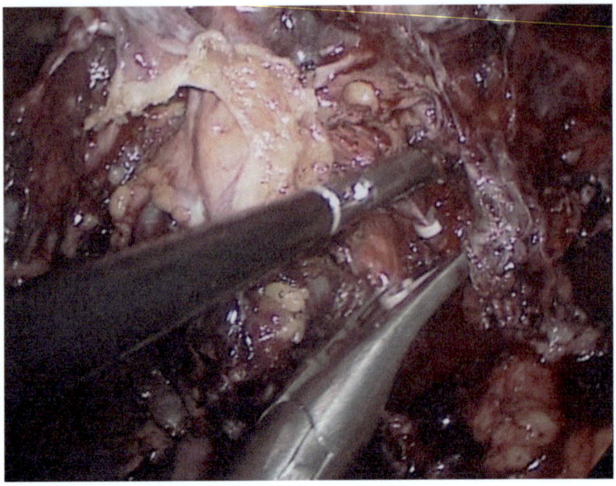

Fig. 4.5 Clamp the vessels in the cystic cavity

diseases, the management should be taken from outer lesions to inner ones. In essence, it is unnecessary to deal with the residual cystic cavity. But in consideration of postoperative adhesion which may lead to the atresia of fenestration, especially in polycystic liver disease and cysts near the diaphragm, the secretory epithelium within the residual cavity should be destroyed by ethanol or argon knife.

4. *Drainage*: When all the cysts have been deroofed and no hemorrhage and bile leak maintained. A draining tube is placed in the cysts cavity. Additional tubes are feasible, if needed. Then insufflation was stopped and trocars are withdrawn. All of the trocar insertion sites should be carefully closed.

4.3 Key Techniques

1. Management of hemorrhage in the cutting edge of cystic wall: Because concomitant bile ducts may exist in most circumstances, the bleeding sites should be clamped by absorbable clip (Fig. 4.5).
2. Management of residual cystic wall: Notice the orientation of hepatic vein and bile duct during the argon plasma coagulation, and the coagulator should be perpendicular to the cystic wall.

4.4 Complications

Although complications of this surgery are rare, there are still reports about hemorrhage and bile leak. With regard to bleeding from the artery, selective arterial embolization or laparoscopic hemostasis should be taken without delay. For bile leak, thorough drainage is needed and percutaneous abdominal puncture drainage by ultrasonic or CT guidance should be conducted if necessary.

4.5 Notes

1. Close observation of patients' examinations and tests
2. Pay attention to variability of drainage's volume and characteristic
3. Patients could have food and drink, activities on the second day after the operation
4. Drainage can be removed, usually 48–72 h postoperatively, if no bleeding and bile leak.
5. Before discharge, an abdominal CT is needed to analyze the residual cystic cavity's status.

Laparoscopic Partial Hepatectomy

5

Abstract

Laparoscopic partial resection or irregular resection of liver tumors are the most undefined type of laparoscopic hepatectomy. Resection of some marginal tumors without major ducts vessels is relatively easy. However, for tumors near the first and second porta hepatis or in segments 7, 8, partial resection is relatively difficult. The overall principle is to keep a distance of at least 1 cm from the edge of the tumor, remove the tumor integrallty, ensure a clean edge, and reduce unnecessary tissue damage.

5.1 Indications and Contraindications

5.1.1 Indications

1. Tumors in segment II, III, IVa, V, VI in Couinaud's segment are best candidates for laparoscopic partial hepatectomy.
2. The size and location of the tumor should not influence the dissection of the first and second porta hepatis. The diameter of tumor should be less than 15 cm in benign cases and 10 cm in malignant cases. Tumor with excessive size limits the operative space and influences the exposure of lesion, in addition, it leaves large cut surface apt to errhysis.
3. The Child-Pugh classification should be at least Grade B, and there should not be any severe structural disease in other organs. The volume of residual liver has to be able to fulfill the physical demand.
4. Patients without complicated upper abdominal operation history, ascites, jaundice, severe cirrhosis, and portal hypertension.
5. Tumor located in liver with intact capsule and without metastasis.

R. Liu, *Laparoscopic Liver Resection*,
https://doi.org/10.1007/978-94-017-9735-1_5

5.1.2 Contraindications

1. Tumor violating inferior vena cava or the root of hepatic vein, which makes the exposure and hemostasis difficult under laparoscopy, is the contradiction of laparoscopic partial hepatectomy.
2. Liver cancer accompanied by intrahepatic metastasis, portal vein tumor thrombus, hilar lymph node metastasis, or unclear tumor boundary is also the contraindication.
3. Patients with complicated upper abdominal operation history and severe intra-abdominal adhesion, ascites, jaundice, severe cirrhosis, and portal hypertension are relative contraindication.
4. Patients with Grade C in Child-Pugh classification or severe dysfunction in other vital organs.
5. Tumor with excessive size interferes the exposure and dissection of first or second porta hepatis.
6. Patients with severe cirrhosis, ascites, jaundice, or hemorrhagic tendency.
7. Patients with poor general condition and unable to withstand major operation and anesthesia.

5.2 Procedure

5.2.1 Patient's Position and Trocar Placement

Patient's position are decided based on the location of the tumor. Typically, the patient is on the supine position. According to the location of the tumor and the habit of surgeons, the 4-trocar technique is usually performed in this procedure. For detailed information, please see Chap. 2.

5.2.2 Laparoscopic Exploration

In combination with imaging examination (Fig. 5.1), laparoscopy is performed to explore the status of liver and other organs, and when the tumor is recognized, its related situation should be assured, such as the location, size, number of tumor, metastasis on the liver surface, enlargement of hilar lymph nodes, adhesion of tumor with surrounding organs, and the degree of cirrhosis (Figs. 5.2 and 5.3). If necessary, especially when the tumor locates deep inside the parenchyma and unable to be seen from the liver surface, intraoperative laparoscopic ultrasonography should be used to detect the location, size, and extent of the hepatic tumor, its relationship to the hepatic vasculature, and to assist the estimation of operation feasibility and selection of proper operation plan with adequate margins.

Wedge resection is suitable for local liver tumor or tumor in the peripheral of liver and sometimes the resection can be extended.

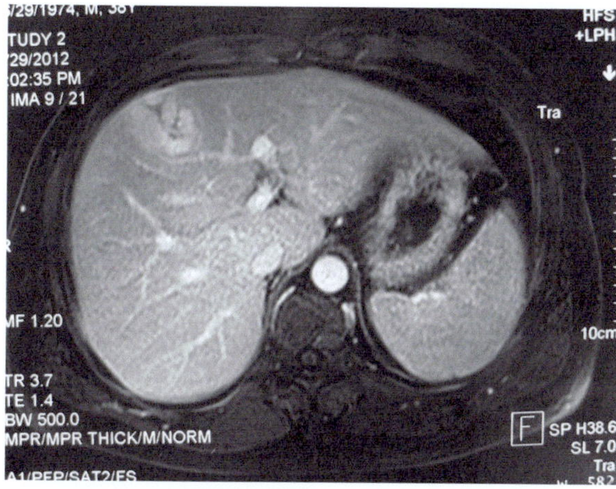

Fig. 5.1 MRI shows the tumor above the gallbladder bed in the right liver

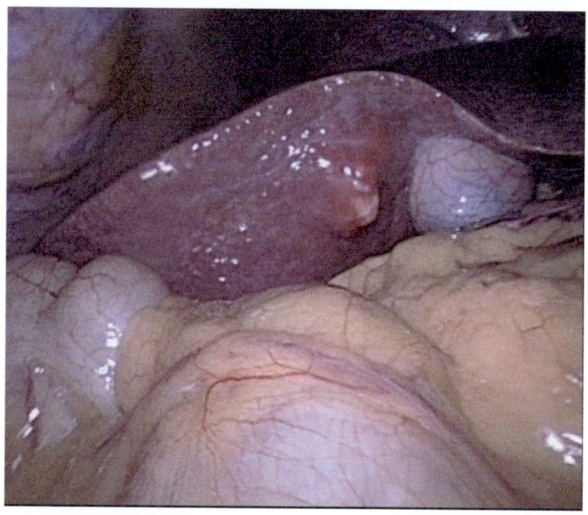

Fig. 5.2 Laparoscopic exploration, the tumor is located in segment 5 and near the gallbladder bed

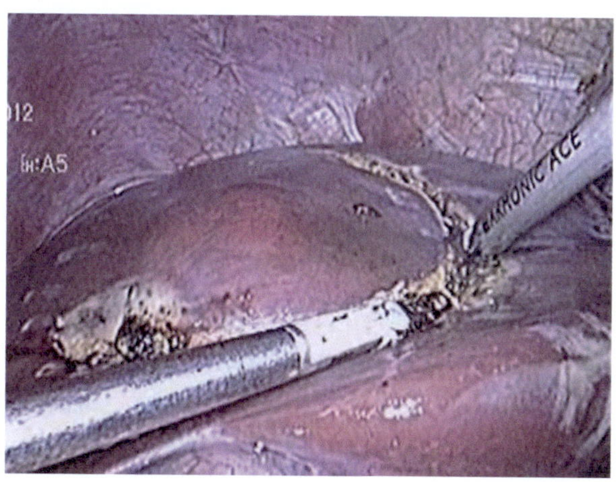

Fig. 5.3 Laparoscopic exploration, the tumor is located in the hepatic diaphragmatic surface

5.2.3 Partial Hepatectomy

For partial resection of small tumors located in the peripheral of right or left liver, technical requirements is undemanding, which doesn't need dissection of the first and second porta hepatis. Based on the different location of tumors, related ligaments transected and part of the liver is dissociated, and a transection plane is outlined on the liver capsule 1–2 cm away from the tumor by electrocoagulator (Fig. 5.4). Then liver parenchyma under the line of transection is dissected by ultrasonic scalpel, during which small hemorrhage can be controlled by mono-polar or bipolar electrocoagulation, while large vessels and bile ducts must be clipped by Hem-o-lock (Figs. 5.5 and 5.6). Attention should be paid to timely flush operative field and aspirate fluid, so as to make the visual filed clean and clear (Fig. 5.7).

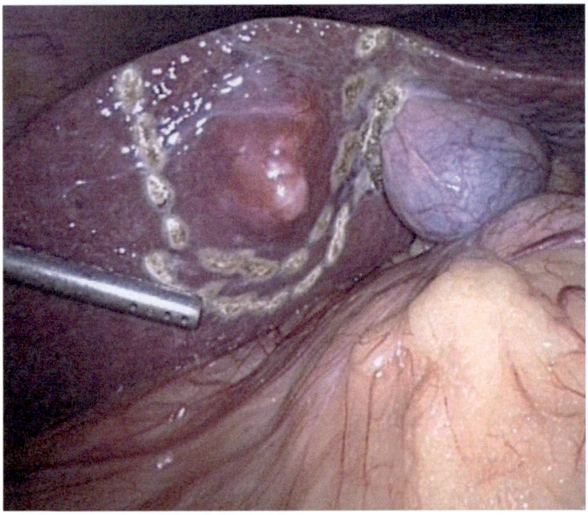

Fig. 5.4 Outline the transection plane on the liver capsule

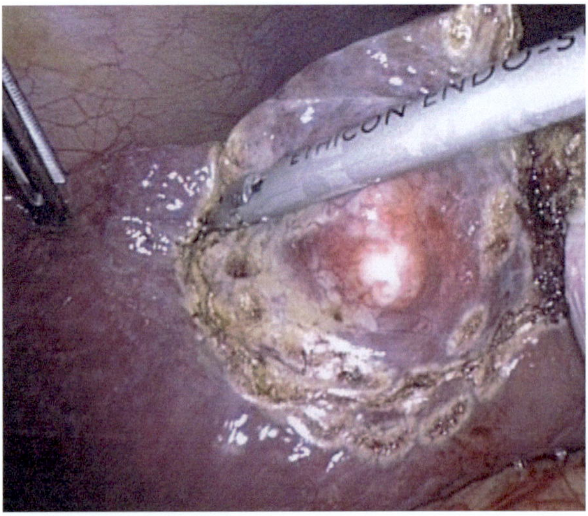

Fig. 5.5 Dissect the liver parenchyma along the pre-set transection plane

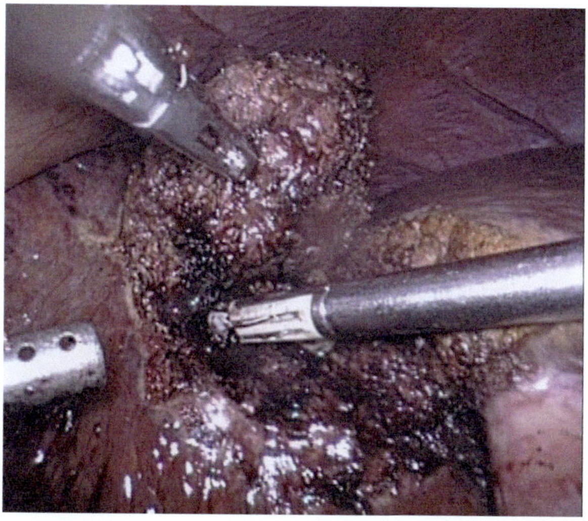

Fig. 5.6 Control the active bleeding using BiClamp forceps

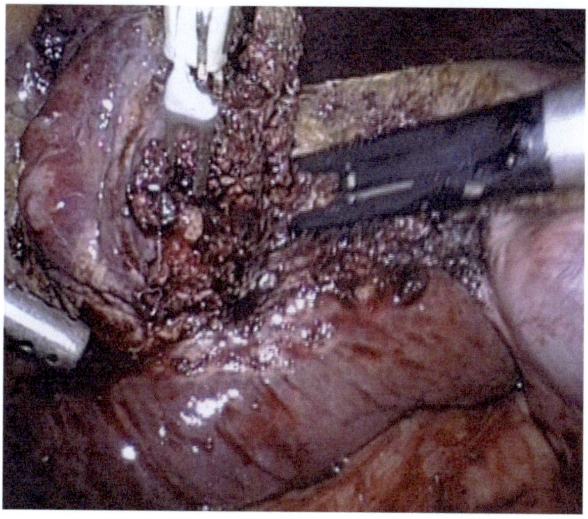

Fig. 5.7 Clamp the inflow vessels using absorbable clip

If tumors located in thin part of liver such as left lateral lobe, wedge transection of liver parenchyma can be carried out by endoscopic linear cutter staplers in a V-shape.

For large-scale partial hepatectomy, the incisional surface is large and the vessels can't be ligated like independent pedicle ligation in anatomic hepatectomy. For the purpose of reducing hemorrhage, familiarity with pre-operative imaging data, especially the enhanced CT or MRI, and performing 3-D reconstruction of the lesion is crucial and may help to decide the main blood supply of tumor. With the help of 3-D reconstruction of tumor supply vessels or guidance by intra-operative ultrasonography when necessary, surgeons dissect liver parenchyma, find and ligate or clip the main supply vessels, and then resect the residual parenchyma. Under the circumstance of massive hemorrhage and unclear vision, it's suggested to press the bleeding point with gauze, resect the tumor fast, and then suture the bleeding vessels.

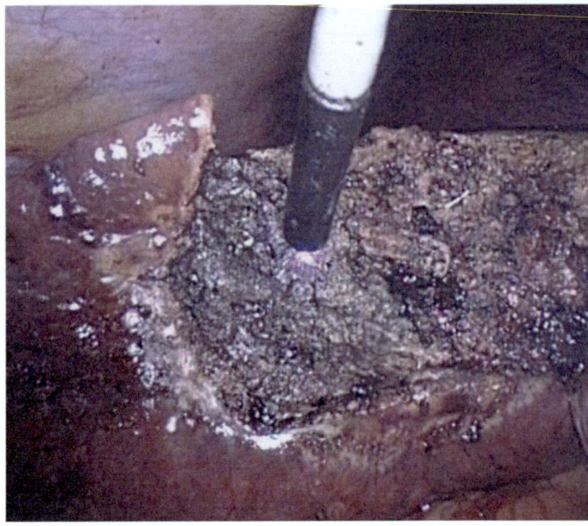

Fig. 5.8 Hemostasis in the cutting edge using argon plasma coagulator

5.2.4 Hemostasis and Drainage

After resection of the lesion, thorough hemostasis of the incisional surface should be achieved by argon beam coagulator or electrocautery (bio electrocoagulator or Biclamp may achieve better hemostasis) (Fig. 5.8), and then biomedical fibrin glue or absorbable hemostatic gauze should be covered on the incisional surface. Whether placing the drainage tube depends on the size of incisional surface and the state of hemostasis. In general, at the last of operation, a fine latex tube is placed through the right trocar and then removed on the first postoperative day if no hemorrhage and biliary fistula occurs. Liver specimen is placed in a plastic bag and extracted from the abdominal cavity through a 3–5 cm enlarged trocar incision (usually under the umbilicus). The liver specimen can also be extracted from posterior fornix in married female patients.

5.3 Major Operating Points

1. Patient position and ports placement is crucial. During the process of ports placement, the feasibility and convenience of the transection line of liver, the dissociation of liver, utilization of endoscopic cutter stapler, extraction of specimen and conversion to laparotomy should also be taken into account.
2. We recommend using the ultrasonic scalpel combined with Biclamp for liver transection and using bipolar and ligasure for electrocoagulation.
3. Make sure a negative margin in malignant tumors.
4. Make a reasonable plan for the transection line of liver.
5. The order of liver transection and hemostasis of incisional surface vary from different types of hemorrhage. Some types of hemorrhage should be stopped immediately while other types be stopped after the resection of lesion.

6. In order to maintain safety, the laparoscopic partial hepatectomy should be conversed to laparotomy timely under certain circumstances: (1) Extensive intra-abdominal adhesions causing difficulty in dissection, severe hemorrhage or rupture of digestive tract. (2) Tumor with large size unable to dissociation, influencing the dissection and exposure of the first and second porta hepatis. (3) Massive hemorrhage unable to be stopped efficiently, especially in cirrhosis patients. Intra-operative bleeding is a critical factor to the prognosis of patients, thus, it's suggested to convert to laparotomy under strict criterion and try not to perform blood transfusion. For benign tumor with relative normal liver function, such as hemangioma, operation can be continued with autologous transfusion. However, blood loss at 800 ml is the alert for conversion, and conversion should be carried out immediately if the operation can't be finished when blood loss at 1200 ml. (4) In case of the injury of extra-hepatic vein trunk unable to be repaired fast (such as clipping the crevasse at once), to avoid CO_2 embolism, surgeons should exhaust intra-abdominal gases and conversion to laparotomy as soon as possible. Be careful to avoid clipping or suturing the crevasse repeatedly, which may enlarge the crevasse and cause serious consequences. (5) Sudden hemorrhage which is unable to be expeditiously controlled, such as bleeding of intrahepatic vein or tumor rupture, should be pressed to control temporarily, and then the surgery should be converted to laparotomy for further operation. (6) During the operation, when the following situations are confirmed, such as liver cancer accompanied by intrahepatic metastasis, portal vein tumor thrombus, hilar lymph node metastasis or unclear tumor territory which may influence the radical principles of malignancy resection, the laparoscopy should be converted to laparotomy.

5.4 Complications

5.4.1 Intra-Operative Hemorrhage

Laparoscopic surgery, in the strict sense, should be a "bloodless" surgery and achieve "hemostasis priority to incision." Once bleeding occurs in laparoscopic surgery, surgeons will lose clear vision immediately, and it's unlikely to clear the blood away and press the bleeding site fast just like in the laparotomy. Therefore, hemorrhage is the most common complication of laparoscopic surgery and the main reason of conversion. Strategies should be taken to prevent hemorrhage in laparoscopic liver resection. For example, surgeons should carefully study the preoperative imaging data, determine the lesion site and the territory of liver resection, so as to make a scientific operation plan. Surgeons should also be careful during operation and avoid damaging large blood vessels. More than that, particular attention should be paid when dissecting the second porta hepatis, and it's advocated to transect hepatic veins inside the liver parenchyma instead of out of the parenchyma.

If an unexpected bleeding occurred during the operation, surgeons must remain calm. The assistant who holds laparoscope should try to maintain the view and keep distant from the bleeding site to avoid the lens shielding by blood. The operator uses the laparoscopic instruments to press the hemorrhage site temporarily to reduce bleeding, during which the assistant aspirates the blood quickly to find out the specific blood site and its origin, and then decides the further appropriate hemostatic method.

1. Hemorrhage from the first porta hepatis: Hemorrhage from branches of the portal vein or hepatic artery, whose color is more vivid, is in a "spewing" or "Jet" shape. As long as operator controls bleeding with left hand and the assistant aspirates the blood, the operator can clip or suture the bleeding site under direct vision with right hand. Sometimes when dissecting one side of the portal vein, small branches of caudate lobe on the posterior wall of portal vein will be tore, which is usually more difficult to deal with. One effective way to dispose that is to keep dissecting the branches of portal vein and then clip or suture the branches. The another method is to insert an absorbable hemostatic gauze or sponge into the posterior of portal vein, press the bleeding site for a few minutes and then continue the operation after the bleeding is controlled. Never blindly clip or electrocoagulate repeatedly in the blood, otherwise there is the risk of injury in the contralateral bile duct.
2. Hemorrhage during liver resection: If the color of blood is vivid, the blood may come from the "infusion vessels," and it can be stopped by bio-polar electrocoagulator. However, when the color of blood is dark and the pressure is low, the blood may come from branches of hepatic veins. In this situation, as the wall of hepatic veins is thin and prone to be tore, absorbable clips should be used to clip both the hepatic vein and its surrounding parenchyma under the bleeding site, instead of lifting up the vessels and then clipping them like in the case of processing portal vein and hepatic artery hemorrhage. In order to prevent gas embolism, the open hepatic vein shouldn't be clipped repeatedly when it's still bleeding. If the bleeding can't be controlled after clipping one to two times, it's suggested to use the gauze to press the bleeding site for a few minutes. For the pressure of hepatic vein is low, the bleeding may ameliorate or stop, and then choose to suture or press the bleeding site based on the actual situation.
3. Hemorrhage from the second porta hepatis: In general, hemorrhage from the second porta hepatis is from the injured hepatic veins or inferior vena cava. If the crevasse is small, the operation can continue after clamping the crevasse with absorbable clip. However, if the crevasse is large, the hemorrhage should be controlled by titanium clip or gauze, and then immediately covert to laparotomy to repair the vessel damage. It's recommended not to suture the hepatic vein under the pneumoperitoneum in laparoscopy, as it may enlarge the crevasse or cause gas embolism.

5.4.2 CO_2 Embolism

Generally,CO_2 embolism occurs when hepatic vein is injured and high pressure CO_2 gets into the heart through venous system, which is one of the most common causes of death in laparoscopic liver resection. Even though many studies have been done on the prevention of CO_2 embolism, there are few effective ways to solve this problem. To prevent CO_2 embolism, it's suggested to dissect the hepatic vein outside of the liver before parenchyma transection and clip the vein with titanium clip. Left and right hepatic vein can both be dissected for 1–2 cm outside of the liver in laparoscopy. But it should be noted that transecting the hepatic vein outside of the liver parenchyma is very dangerous. If disposing inappropriately, it may lead to the death of patient in a short time. In laparoscopic left lateral lobectomy, there's no need to dissect left hepatic vein outside of the liver parenchyma.

5.4.3 Biliary Fistula

In the process of parenchyma transection, sometimes it may occur to bile leak. After clearing the intra-abdominal operative area, use a dry gauze to wipe the incisional surface so as to check whether bile leak exists. If the leak comes from the cut end of bile duct, it needs to be clipped or sutured. However, when the bile leak is from the crevasse of bile duct in the residual liver, the crevasse needs to be repaired by fine needle. Referring to the post-operative biliary fistula, when the volume of bile leak is limited, the fistula can be healed by keeping the drainage tube fluent. However, when the volume of bile leak is large or the bile diffuses among the abdominal cavity, laparoscopic or open exploration should be carried out to ascertain the status of biliary fistula and then dispose the fistula.

5.5 Notes

1. Closely observe vital signs of patients after the surgery.
2. Pay attention to the volume and property of drainage fluid.
3. Sustain the balance of water, electrolyte, and acid–base metabolism.
4. Remove the nasogastric decompression tube 6 h after the surgery, give the patients fluid diet and then normal diet gradually.

6 Laparoscopic Single-Site Hepatectomy

Abstract

With the improvement of laparoscopic instruments and surgical experience, significant development has been gained in laparoscopic liver surgery. However, it is still the dream of both surgeons and patients to reduce the surgical injury to the maximum extent. In recent years, laparoscopic single-site surgery has been constantly tried as a new challenging technique. Laparoscopic single-site hepatectomy may play a promising role in the field of the minimally invasive surgery.

With the improvement of laparoscopic instruments and surgical experience, significant development has been gained in laparoscopic liver surgery. However, it is still the dream of both surgeons and patients to reduce the surgical injury to the maximum extent. In recent years, laparoscopic single-site surgery has been constantly tried as a new challenging technique. Laparoscopic single-site hepatectomy may play a promising role in the field of the minimally invasive surgery.

6.1 Indications

1. Malignant tumor, diameter ≤2.5 cm; or benign tumor, diameter ≤5 cm.
2. Lesions located in the segments 3 & 4b, protruding from the surface of the liver.
3. No morbid obesity; No history of upper abdominal surgery (Fig. 6.1).

6.2 Steps and Key Techniques

1. Patient is in the reverse Trendelenburg position with two legs apart, general intravenous anesthesia, mechanical ventilation with laryngeal mask or endotracheal intubation. The surgeon stands on the middle, and the assistants on the sides of the surgeon (Figs. 6.2 and 6.3).

R. Liu, *Laparoscopic Liver Resection*,
https://doi.org/10.1007/978-94-017-9735-1_6

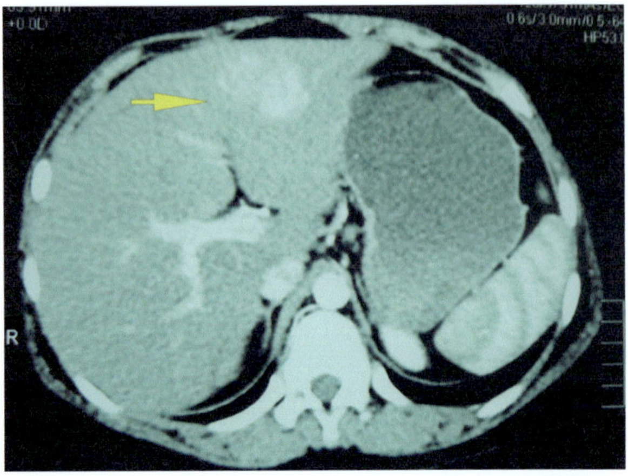

Fig. 6.1 Focal nodular hyperplasia (FNH) located in Segment 3

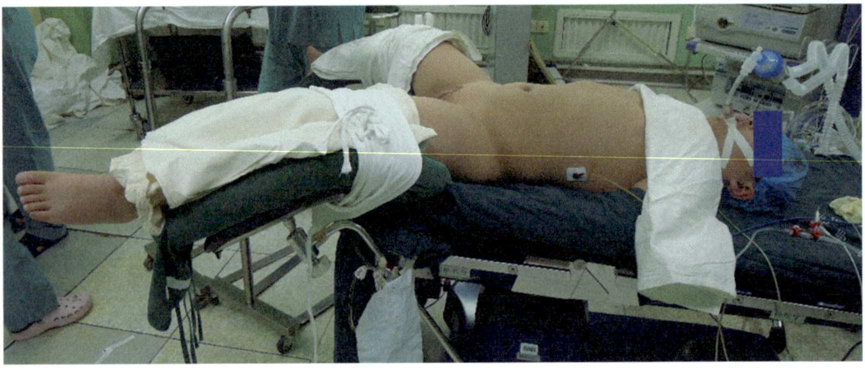

Fig. 6.2 Position of the patient

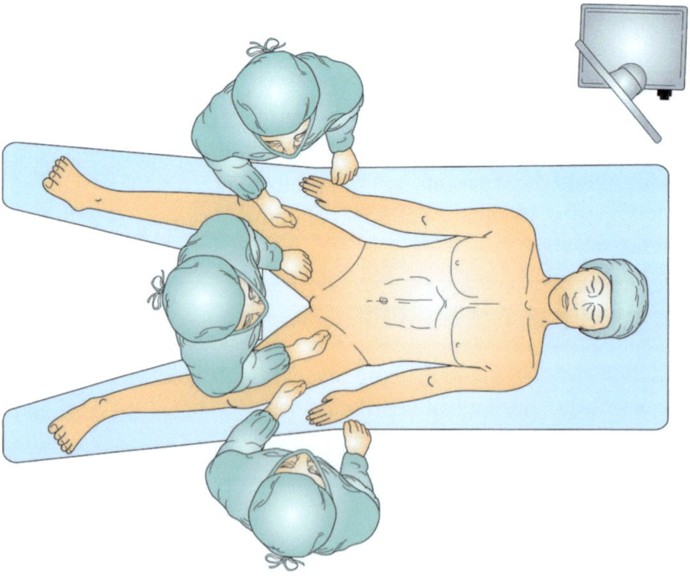

Fig. 6.3 Position of surgeons

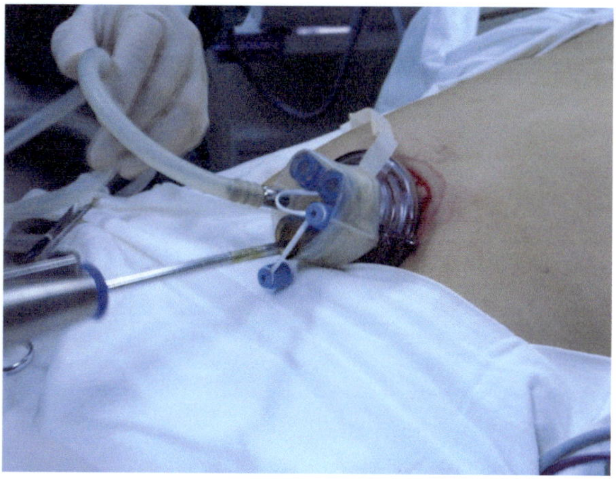

Fig. 6.4 The Triport access

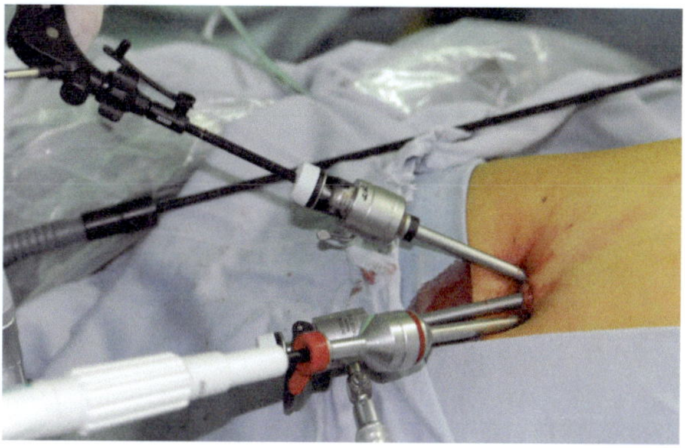

Fig. 6.5 The three 5 mm trocars' access

2. The Triport is, or three adjacent 5 mm transumbilical trocars are used to build the access through the abdominal wall; the 30° bendable 5 mm laparoscope; other laparoscopic instruments include dissecting forceps, grasping forceps and scissors, endoscopic linear staples, harmonic scalpel, Biclamp and LigaSure (Figs. 6.4 and 6.5).
3. The long-distance laparoscopic observation at most time. When a magnifying vision is needed, the laparoscope is adjusted firstly and then the other surgical instruments; endoscopic linear staples with joint are more preferable.
4. Other than harmonic scalpel resection alone, the wedge resection can also be performed by two crossed endoscopic linear staples (Figs. 6.6 and 6.7).
5. Postoperative drainage (Fig. 6.8)

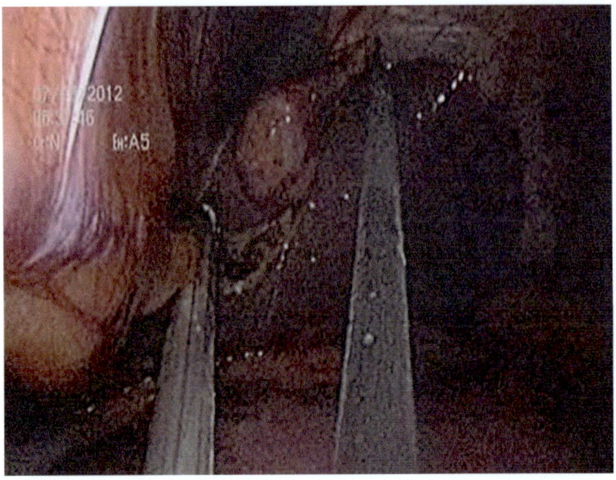

Fig. 6.6 Hepatectomy by harmonic scalpel

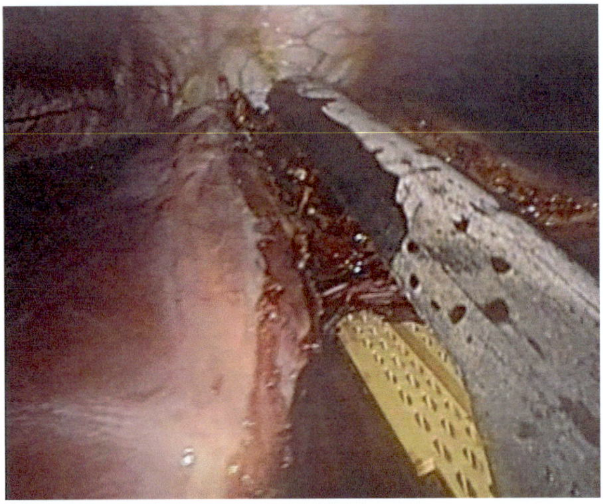

Fig. 6.7 Hepatectomy by endoscopic linear staples

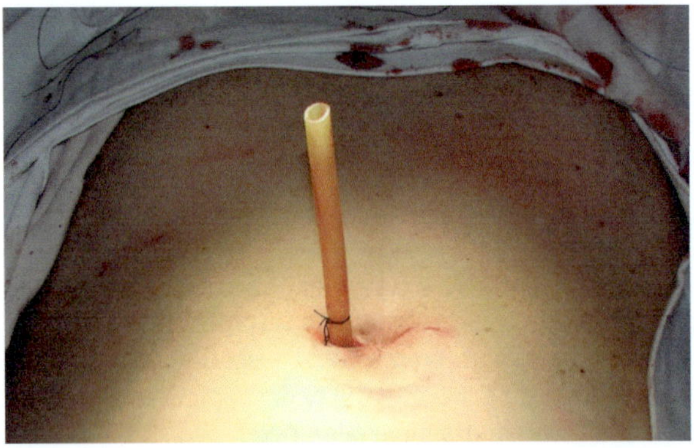

Fig. 6.8 Transumbilical postoperative drainage

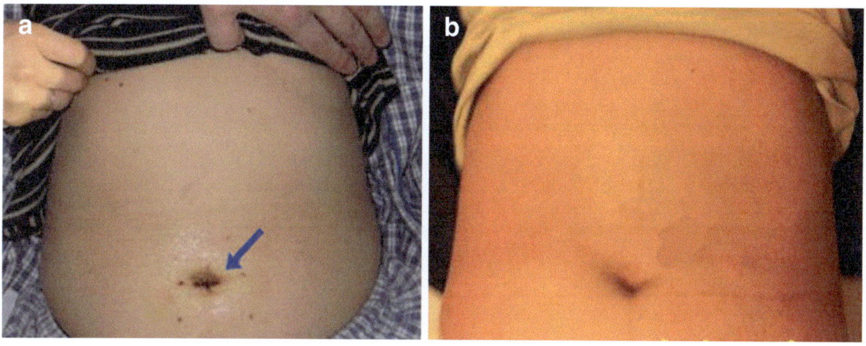

Fig. 6.9 The comparison of incisions of the laparoscopic single-site hepatectomy: (**a**) 1 day after surgery; (**b**) 4 weeks after surgery

6.3 Advantages

Laparoscopic single-site hepatectomy can reduce the injury of the abdominal wall and subsequent postoperative pain. Its obvious scarless characteristic can meet the cosmetic needs of patients (Fig. 6.9).

6.4 Disadvantages

1. Laparoscopic instruments remain to be improved: There are no specialized laparoscopic single-site dissecting forceps or linear staples. The single-site laparoscopic instrument should be able to rotate by multiangles with a sufficient length to avoid the mutual interference. To use the conventional instruments for laparoscopic single-site surgery is difficult to cope with the complex surgeries or difficult situation such as massive bleeding.
2. Laparoscopic lens remains to be improved: The 5 mm lens gets less light through and results in an unclear gloomy surgical field.
3. To remove the specimen, the abdominal incision often need be expanded. The oversized incision may make single-site surgery meaningless. In this case, the new approach, such as vaginal formix, may be considered.

6.5 Notes

1. Extra conscious should be paid to prevent the blockage of the drainage tube.
2. Cases should be performed with a strict inclusion criteria, and conversion to mutiple-trocar method or even open procedure should be concerned if necessary.

Laparoscopic Left Lateral Sectionectomy

7

Abstract

Left lateral section contains the segments 2 and 3. The unique anatomical structure of the left lateral section makes laparoscopic left lateral sectionectomy (LLLS) one of the most applied laparoscopic liver resection surgeries. With almost the same or even shorted operation time, LLLS has the advantages such as smaller incision and less injuries. The short-term prognosis of LLLS is significantly better than that of open surgery. According to our own experience, we brought up a practical method called "Seven-step liver transection."

Left lateral section contains the segments 2 and 3. The unique anatomical structure of the left lateral section makes laparoscopic left lateral sectionectomy (LLLS) one of the most applied laparoscopic liver resection surgeries. With almost the same or even shorted operation time, LLLS has the advantages such as smaller incision and less injuries. The short-term prognosis of LLLS is significantly better than that of open surgery. According to our own experience, we brought up a practical method called "Seven-step liver transection."

7.1 Indications and Contraindications

7.1.1 Indications

1. Benign or malignant tumor located limitedly in the left lateral section; No limit for the size of the tumor only if porta hepatis available.
2. Intrahepatic bile duct stones with a left atrophy lateral section.
3. Liver function of Child B or better
4. No history of complex abdominal surgery

R. Liu, *Laparoscopic Liver Resection*,
https://doi.org/10.1007/978-94-017-9735-1_7

7.1.2 Contraindications

1. General contraindications, such as metastatic lesions or adjacent organ infiltration;
2. Lymphadenectomy is needed for the metastatic lymphatic lesions. Embolectomy is needed for the cancer thrombus in the bile duct, portal vein or inferior vena cava;
3. Compression or infiltration to the first or second porta hepatis;
4. History of complex abdominal surgery;
5. The general condition is too poor to tolerate pneumoperitoneum or general anesthesia.

7.2 Steps

7.2.1 Patient Position and Trocar Distribution

The supine position and intubated intravenous anesthesia are adopted. The four-trocar method is taken. The main and auxiliary 12 mm operation trocars are placed on the subcostal left and right side of the rectus abdominis respectively. The assistant 5 mm trocar is located beneath the left main operation trocar with the interval of at least 5 cm. See Chap. 2.

7.2.2 Exploration and Mobilization

After a comprehensive exploration of the abdominal organs, the location and size of the tumor should be assessed meticulously (Figs. 7.1 and 7.2). The perihepatic ligaments are transected by harmonic scalpel from round ligament, falciform ligament, left coronary ligament to left deltoid ligament in turn. The lesser omentum is transected with harmonic scalpel until the root of the ligamentum venosum with the left lateral section lifted by the assistant.

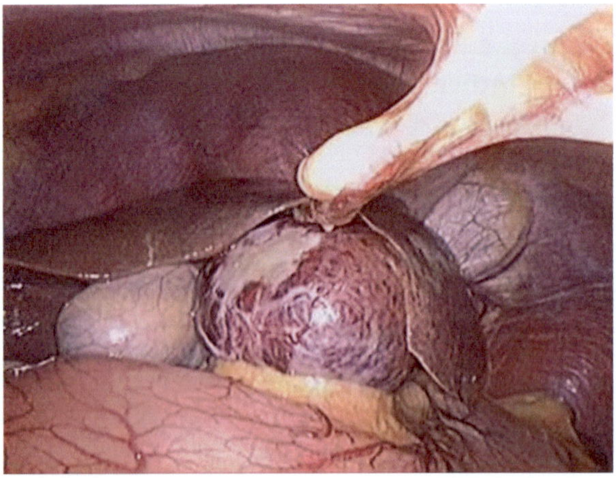

Fig. 7.1 Laparoscopic exploration: a giant hemangioma located in left lateral section

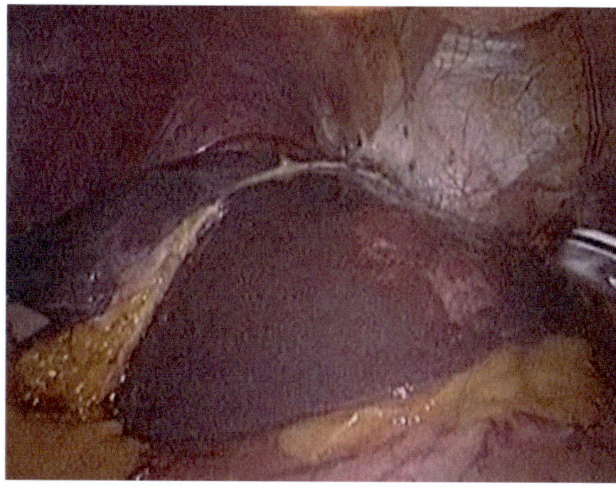

Fig. 7.2 Laparoscopic exploration: a hepatocellular carcinoma located in left lateral section

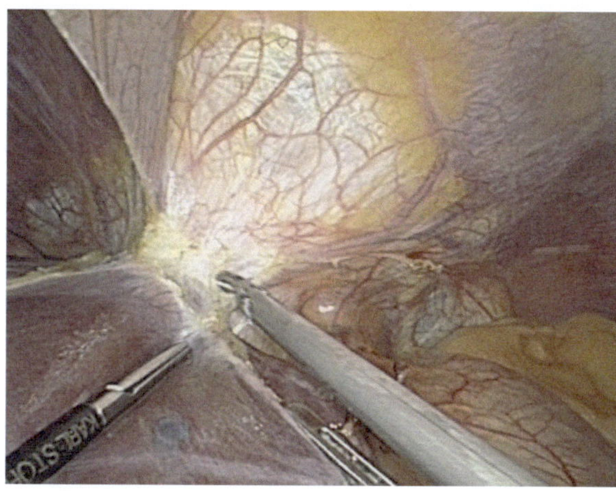

Fig. 7.3 Transection of the left coronary ligament

The round ligament can be transected directly by harmonic scalpel or LigaSure, without ligation of the both stumps. The transection should be close to the abdominal wall. This will help the traction of the liver from the near end without disturbance from the far end.

The second porta hepatis will be exposed after dissection of the suprahepatic ligament. The left inferior phrenic vein drains into the IVC-near right margin of the left coronary ligament, which should be carefully dissected in case of injury.

The transection of the left coronary ligament should start from the middle part and move to the two sides. The over traction of the left deltoid ligament during transection may cause the injury on the diaphragm. The resection line should be close to the liver (Figs. 7.3 and 7.4).

The left lateral section should be drawn to the cranial and lateral direction when the less omentum is dissected. The less omentum should be transected completely in order to introduce the staple passing the visceral surface of the liver (Fig. 7.5).

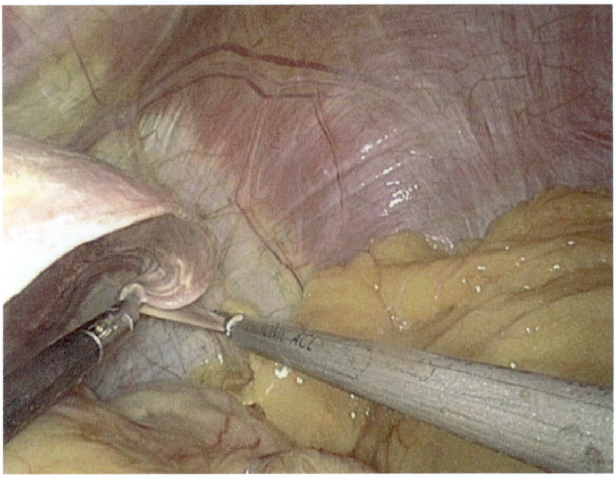

Fig. 7.4 Transection of the left deltoid ligament

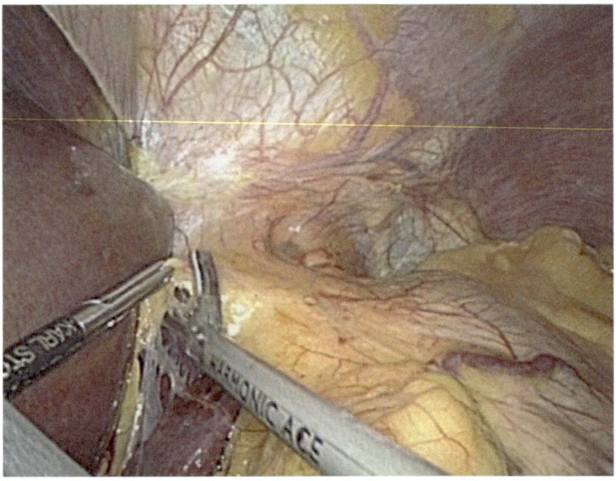

Fig. 7.5 Transection of the less omentum

7.2.3 Rough Dissection of the Portal Pedicles of Segments 2 and 3

The "vessel-less" parenchyma around the portal pedicles of the segments 2 and 3 are roughly dissected to expose the pedicles. Once the linear staple could be used, the dissection should stop (Fig. 7.6).

7.2.4 Transection of the Portal Pedicles of Segments 2 and 3

The linear staple is introduced from the right auxiliary 12 mm trocar and the portal pedicles of the segments 2 and 3 are then transected including the adhesive liver parenchyma. This operation should be performed under direct vision to make sure the entire portal pedicles of the segments 2 and 3 are transected (Fig. 7.7).

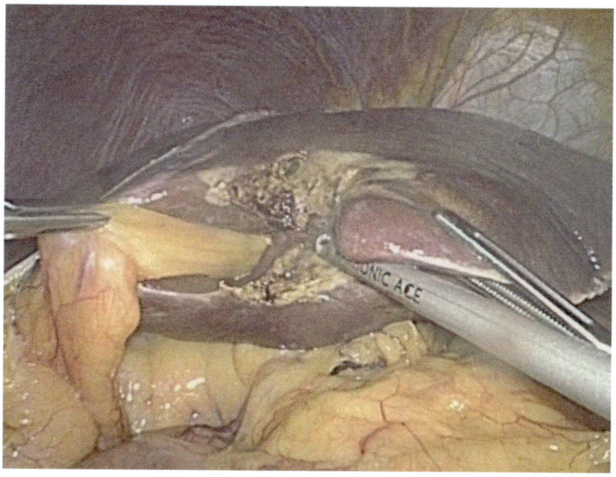

Fig. 7.6 The rough dissection of the portal pedicles of the segments 2 and 3

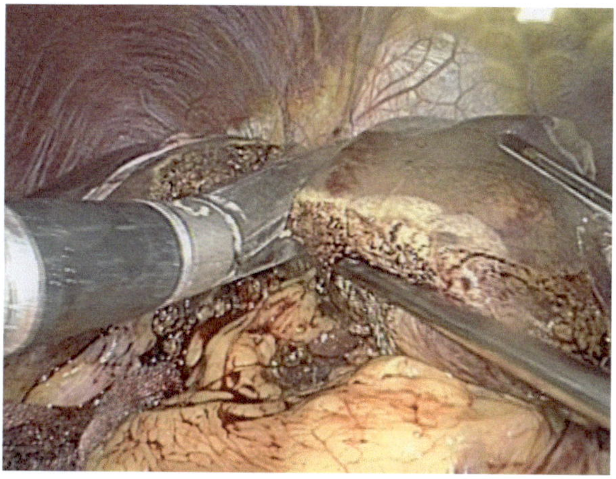

Fig. 7.7 The transection of the portal pedicles of the segments 2 and 3

7.2.5 Dissection of the Deep Parenchyma to Expose LHV

The parenchyma around the LHV are roughly dissected until the staple can contain the remnant liver tissue including the root of the LHV (Fig. 7.8).

7.2.6 Transection of the Left Hepatic Vein

The stump of left deltoid ligament is grasped by the assistant to the anterior and inferior direction. The two tips of the staple should be exposed to make sure the LHV is transected entirely. The LHV is transected including the adhesive liver parenchyma. The injury of the diaphragm and the IVC should be avoided by the staples (Fig. 7.9).

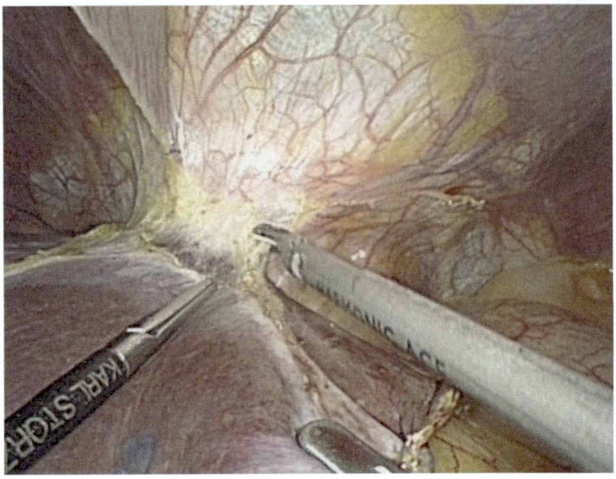

Fig. 7.8 Dissection of the deep parenchyma to expose the LHV

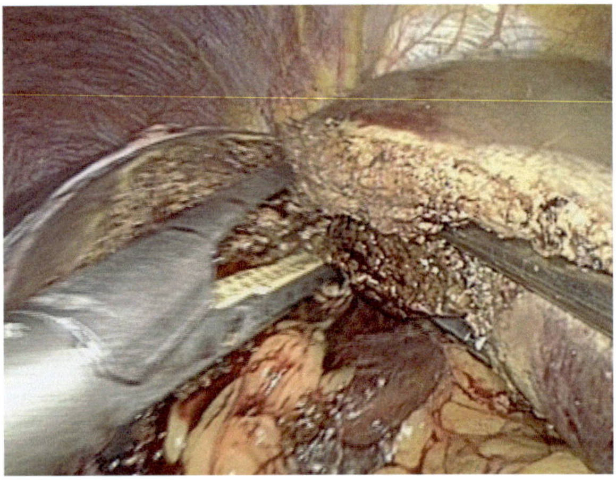

Fig. 7.9 Transection of the left hepatic vein

When the LHV is not totally transected, an absorbable clip should be used to clamp the stump of the LHV. Then the residual tissue could be dissected by scissors or harmonic scalpel. The metal nails in the staple might damage the harmonic scalpel (Fig. 7.10).

7.2.7 Hemostasis and Drainage

The argon beam is used for errhysis of the raw surface. The Biclamp is used for gentle active bleeding. The absorbable clips are used for obvious active bleeding. The suture is used for bile leak and the bleeding impossible to be controlled by other means (Figs. 7.11 and 7.12).

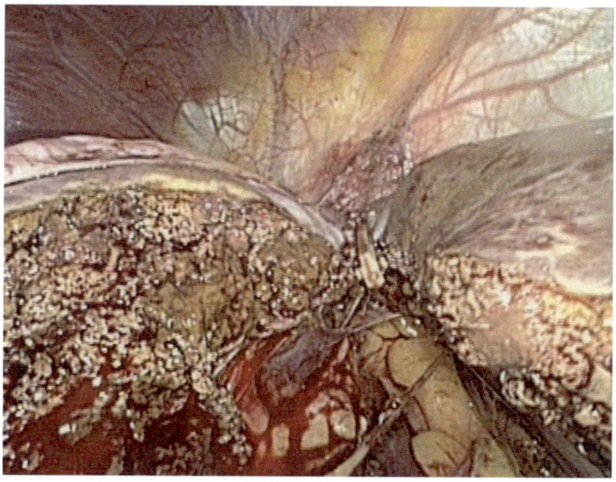

Fig. 7.10 The LHV is not totally transected

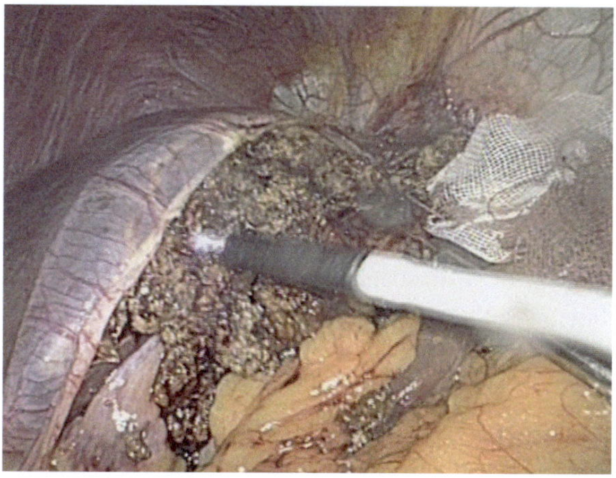

Fig. 7.11 The argon beam for errhysis

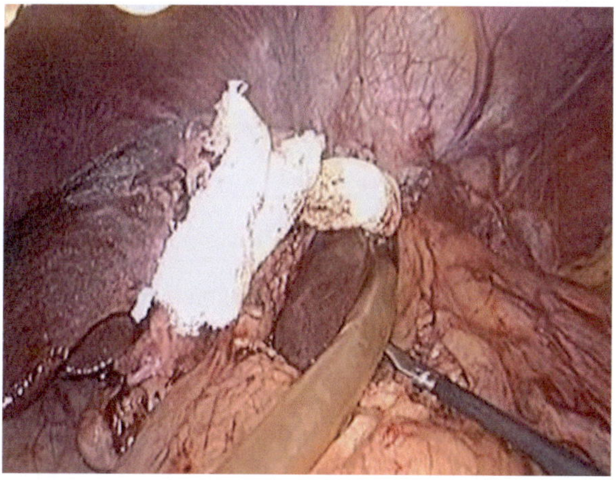

Fig. 7.12 Postoperative drainage

7.2.8 To Withdraw Specimen

The benign tumor specimen could be withdrawn from the expanded umbilical incision after fragmentation. The malignant specimen should be withdrawn as a whole in case of possible dissemination. There are four approaches to withdraw the specimen: (a) through the incision between the main and auxiliary operational holes; (b) through the scar of the previous surgery; (c) through a new incision above the symphysis pubis; (d) through the vaginal fornix incision.

7.3 Key Techniques

1. The intraoperative vascular occlusion and dissection of the LHV are needless.
2. The full mobilization of the lateral liver section is the key for the safe use of the staple.
3. The portal pedicles of the segments 2 and 3 are roughly dissected.
4. The dissection line of the deep parenchyma to expose the LHV should be a little bit to the left so that the LHV could be ligated entirely.

7.4 Complications

1. The intraoperative and postoperative complications can be managed similarly to those of laparoscopic partial hepatectomy.
2. For the arteries and portal bleeding, "the three-step hemostasis method" could be used after the control of the vision by the suction and compression of the gauze. Firstly, the Biclamp is used to coagulate. Secondly, the absorbable clip, titanium clip or Hem-o-lok is used on the target vessel. Thirdly, laparoscopic suture is the last step before conversion.
3. The hepatic vein bleeding should be managed with great caution to avoid gas embolism. For partial hepatic vein fracture, the clip or staple is preferable. When the stump of the hepatic vein has shrunk into the liver parenchyma, the coagulation may not work. After the control of the vision by the suction and gauze, the surgeon should try to grasp the stump and then use the clip or suture to fix the fracture. The repeating trying in a short time is not wise.

7.5 Notes

1. The gastrointestinal decompression and ureteral catheterization can stop on the first postoperative day. The patient can intake liquid diet. After 3–5 days, the patient can be discharged.
2. The second surgery can also be performed laparoscopically for the uncontrollable postoperative abdominal bleeding.

Laparoscopic Left Hepatectomy

8

Abstract

Left semi-liver contains the segments 2, 3, and 4. There are some similarities between laparoscopic and open left hepatectomy. They both belong to the anatomic liver resection. They both need dissection of the first hilum to control the inflow blood. However, the outflow of the hepatic vein can be difficult to occlude in an extra-hepatic way before the parenchyma dissection laparoscopically. It also could be transected along with the parenchyma dissection. Laparoscopic left hepatectomy is still challenging and demanding surgery.

Left semi-liver contains the segments 2, 3, and 4. There are some similarities between laparoscopic and open left hepatectomy. They both belong to the anatomic liver resection. They both need dissection of the first hilum to control the inflow blood. However, the outflow of the hepatic vein can be difficult to occlude in an extra-hepatic way before the parenchyma dissection laparoscopically. It also could be transected along with the parenchyma dissection. Laparoscopic left hepatectomy is still challenging and demanding surgery.

8.1 Indications and Contraindications

8.1.1 Indications

1. Lesion located limitedly in the segments 2, 3, and 4 while less resection is inappropriate.
2. The first and second porta hepatis could be manipulated. Malignant tumor, diameter ≤10 cm; or benign tumor, diameter ≤15 cm.
3. Liver function of Child B or better
4. Donor of the living liver transplantation

R. Liu, *Laparoscopic Liver Resection*,
https://doi.org/10.1007/978-94-017-9735-1_8

8.1.2 Contraindications

1. Compression or infiltration to the first or second porta hepatis;
2. Lymphadenectomy is needed for the metastatic lymphatic lesions. Embolectomy is needed for the cancer thrombus in the bile duct, portal vein or inferior vena cava;
3. History of complex abdominal surgery;
4. The general condition is too poor to tolerate pneumoperitoneum or general anesthesia.

8.2 Steps

8.2.1 Patient Position and Trocar Distribution

The supine position is taken. The operational table should be adjusted according to the intraoperative needs. See Chap. 2 for trocar distribution.

8.2.2 Exploration and Mobilization

After a comprehensive exploration of the abdominal organs, the location and size of the tumor should be assessed meticulously. The key points of the tumor include location, size, number, possible metastasis lesions and the level of liver cirrhosis. The laparoscopic ultrasonography will help to decide the resectability and alternative surgical plans.

The order to mobilize left semi-liver is round ligament, falciform ligament, left coronary ligament and part of right coronary ligament, left deltoid ligament, and then hepatogastric ligament.

The left part of the right coronary ligament should be incised to make the right turn-over of the left semi-liver possible to access (Fig. 8.1).

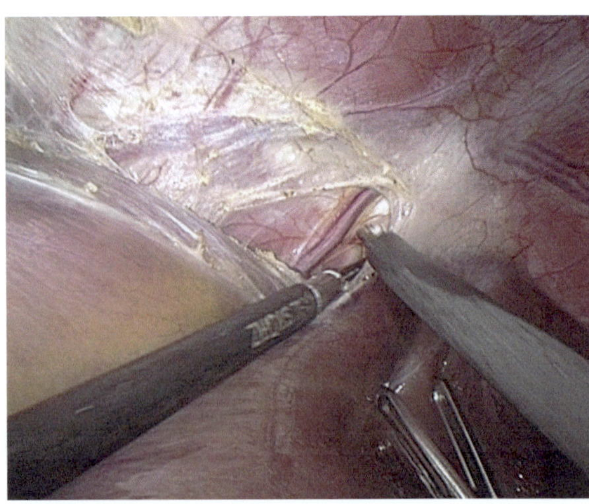

Fig. 8.1 The left part of the right coronary ligament is incised

8.2.3 Dissection of First Hilum and Control of Inflow Blood

The left liver artery can be dissected out by the intra-fascial approach. The right posterior artery originating from the left liver artery should be noticed. The dissection should be close to the liver parenchyma to the maximum extent. Through the Glissonean pedicle approach, the left liver artery and portal vein can be transected at the same time (Figs. 8.2 and 8.3). We usually transect the left portal pedicles after dissection of the superficial liver parenchyma (Figs. 8.4 and 8.5) (see Sect. 8.2.5).

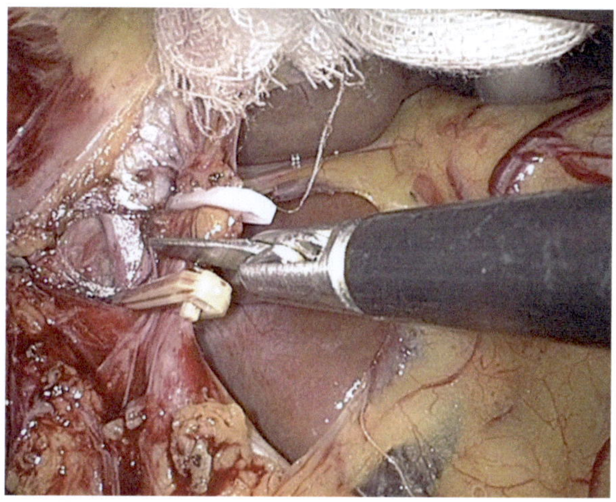

Fig. 8.2 Dissection of the left liver artery (The hilar access approach)

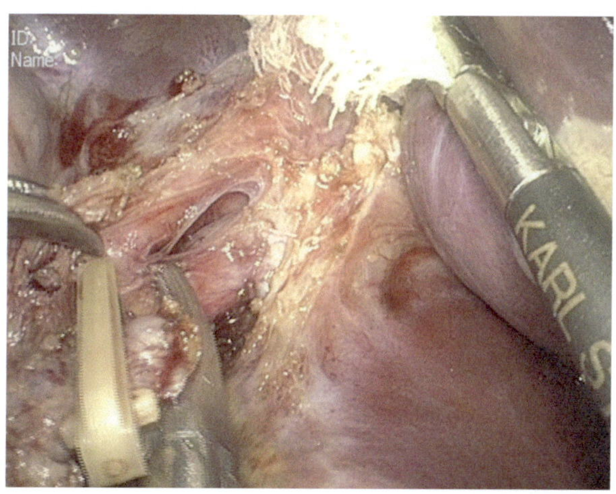

Fig. 8.3 Dissection of the left portal vein (The hilar access approach)

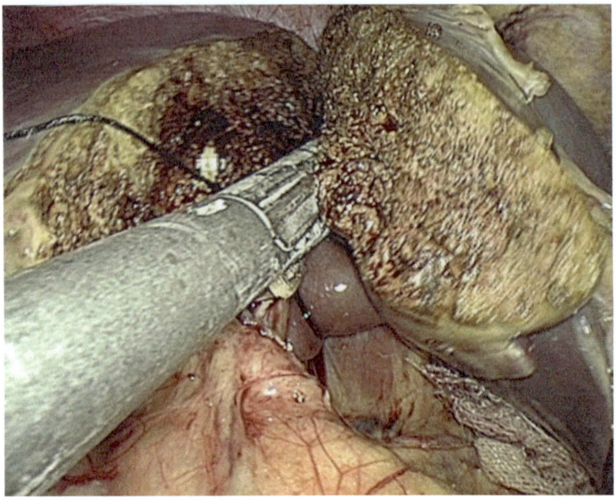

Fig. 8.4 Transection of the left portal pedicles by staple

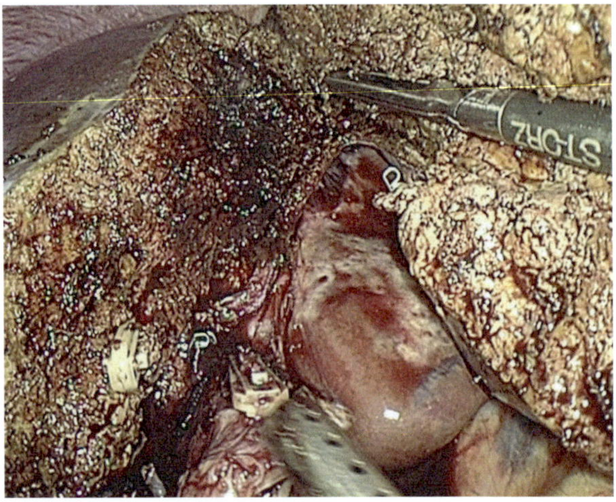

Fig. 8.5 After transection of the left portal pedicles

8.2.4 Exposure of Second Hilum and Control of Outflow Blood

For minor hepatectomy, the LHV should be dissected out without ligation (Fig. 8.6). For major hepatectomy, the LHV should be ligated without transection, mainly considering the possible bleeding from the hepatic vein.

8.2.5 Parenchymal Dissection

According to the ischemic demarcation (Fig. 8.7), the liver parenchyma is dissected by harmonica scalpel and linear staple (Fig. 8.8). The Biclamp and clips are used against bleeding from the cutting. The titanium clip should be avoided, because the occlusal strength is less than the other advanced clips (Fig. 8.9). The dysfunction of the titanium clip may cause unnecessary bleeding. Meanwhile, its existence may have an inconvenient effect on the subsequent operation.

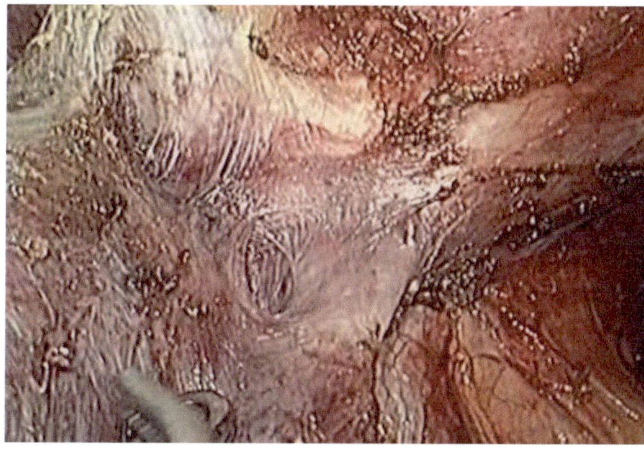

Fig. 8.6 Exposure of the LHV

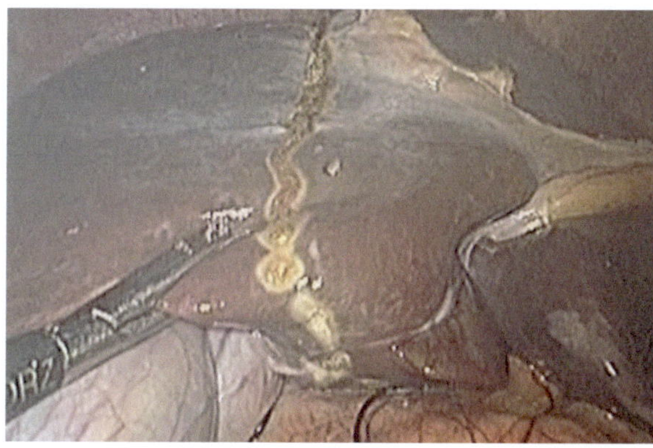

Fig. 8.7 The ischemic line of the liver surface

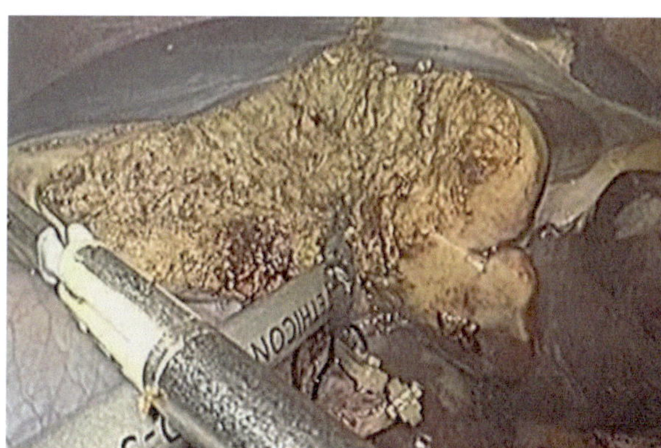

Fig. 8.8 The superficial parenchyma is dissected by harmonic scalpel

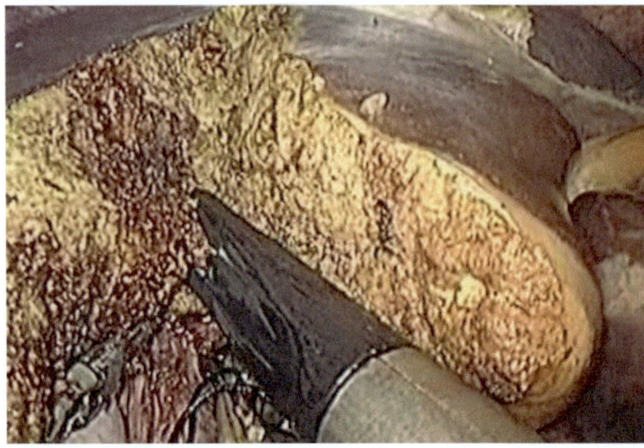

Fig. 8.9 The absorbable chip for the vessels in raw surface

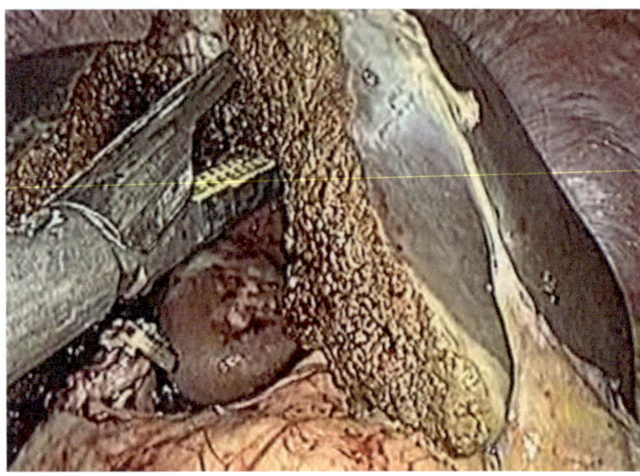

Fig. 8.10 Transection of the LHV

8.2.6 Transection of LHV

The angle and direction of the staple should be carefully chosen when the LHV is transected. The direction of the staple should point to the root of the LHV, even slightly left when necessary, so as to avoid the injury of the MHV (Fig. 8.10). The preoperative images should be thoroughly studied to clarify the relationship between the LHV and MHV. The two tips of the staple should be exposed in vision to avoid the diaphragm injury.

When the LHV is not totally transected, an absorbable clip should be used to clamp the stump of the LHV (Fig. 8.11).

8.2.7 Hemostasis

The argon beam is used for errhysis of the raw surface (Fig. 8.12). The Biclamp is used for gentle active bleeding. The absorbable clips are used for obvious active

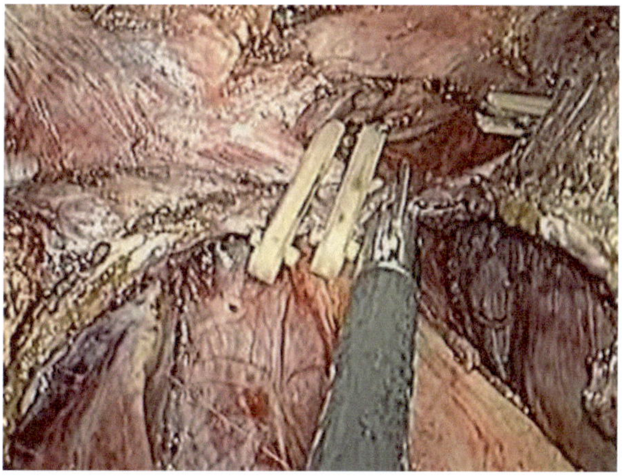

Fig. 8.11 Management of partial transection of the LHV

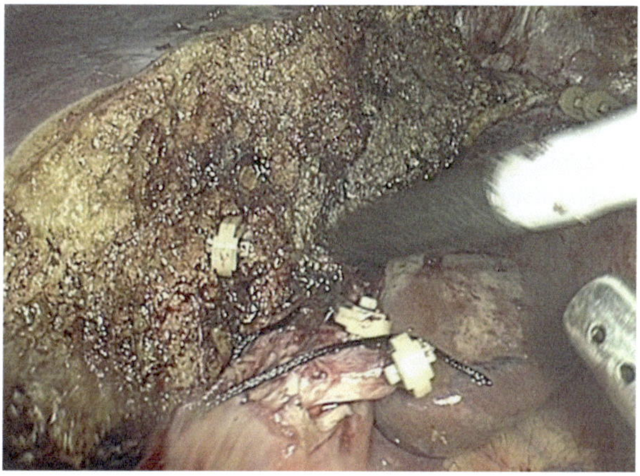

Fig. 8.12 Hemostasis in the raw surface

bleeding. The suture is used for bile leak and the bleeding impossible to be controlled by other means.

8.2.8 To Withdraw Specimen

The specimen is withdrawn with an endoscopic retriever through the expanded incision. It should be inspected immediately.

8.2.9 Drainage

The drainage tube is placed on the raw surface of the liver (Fig. 8.13).

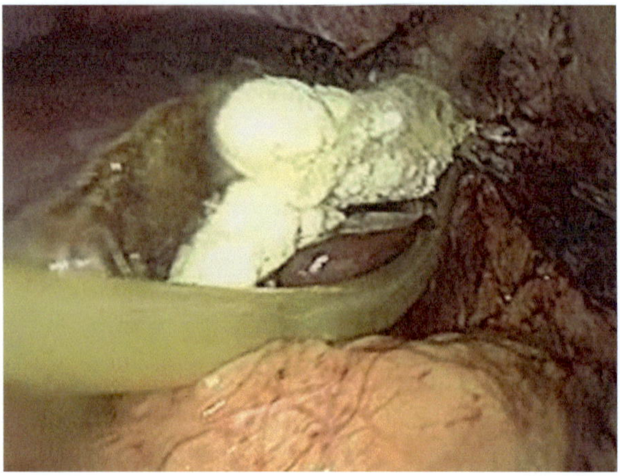

Fig. 8.13 Drainage

8.3 Key Techniques

1. The main operational trocar should be placed carefully. It should not only be convenient for the mobilization and parenchyma transection, but also make the staple through the trocar easy to point along the planned liver cutting plane.
2. The liver should be fully mobilized, especially for the hepatogastric ligament. The hepatogastric ligament should be transected from the root of the LHV to the foramen of Winslow. This will help the exposure of the LHV and introduction of the staple to transect the left portal pedicles.
3. To avoid the injury of the MHV, the direction of the staple should point to the root of the LHV, even slightly left when necessary.
4. When the intraoperative bleeding is over 800 ml, conversion to open surgery should be taken immediately.

8.4 Complications

The intraoperative and postoperative complications can be managed similarly to those of laparoscopic lateral sectionectomy. Also see discussion in Chap. 1.

8.5 Notes

1. The gastrointestinal decompression and ureteral catheterization can stop on the first postoperative day. The patient can intake liquid diet. After 3–5 days, the patient can be discharged.
2. The second surgery can also be performed laparoscopically for the uncontrollable postoperative abdominal bleeding.

9 Laparoscopic Right Posterior Sectionectomy

Abstract

Right posterior section contains the segments 6 and 7. The portal pedicles of the right posterior section can be easily dissected out, because they lie superficially in the right fissure of the hilum.

Right posterior section contains the segments 6 and 7. The portal pedicles of the right posterior section can be easily dissected out, because they lie superficially in the right fissure of the hilum.

9.1 Indications and Contraindications

9.1.1 Indications

1. Lesion located limitedly in the segments 6 and 7 while less resection is inappropriate.
2. The first and second porta hepatis could be manipulated. Malignant tumor, diameter ≤10 cm; or benign tumor, diameter ≤15 cm.
3. Liver function of Child B or better.
4. No portal thrombus; No intrahepatic or systemic metastasis.

9.1.2 Contraindications

1. The invasion to the IVC or the root of RHV;
2. Lymphadenectomy is needed for the metastatic lymphatic lesions. Embolectomy is needed for the cancer thrombus in the bile duct, portal vein or inferior vena cava;
3. History of complex abdominal surgery;
4. The general condition is too poor to tolerate pneumoperitoneum or general anesthesia

R. Liu, *Laparoscopic Liver Resection*,
https://doi.org/10.1007/978-94-017-9735-1_9

9.2 Steps

9.2.1 Patient Position and Trocar Distribution

The left lateral position is taken. The operational table should be adjusted according to the intraoperative needs. See Chap. 2 for trocar distribution.

9.2.2 Exploration

Laparoscopic abdominal exploration is performed comprehensively and combined with the preoperative imaging (Fig. 9.1). The location, size, and number of the tumor should be inspected meticulously. The laparoscopic ultrasonography could further provide the information such as the main feeding vessels of the tumor, existence of the satellite focus, and accurate boundaries of the tumor.

9.2.3 Mobilization

The right perihepatic ligament should be dissected as much as possible (Fig. 9.2). The ligament of left vena cava should also be transected for the convenience of lifting the right section during the surgery.

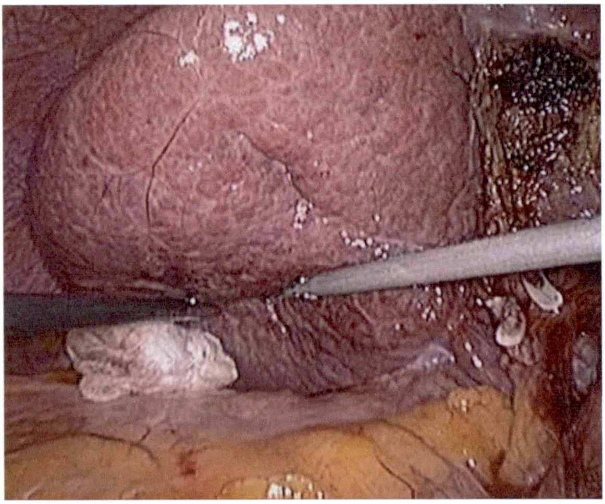

Fig. 9.1 Exploration of the right posterior section

9.2.4 Dissection and Control of Inflow Blood

There is no visible boundary of the right posterior section on the surface of the liver (Fig. 9.3). Identification of the right posterior portal pedicle is the key to perform sectionectomy safely (Fig. 9.3). Once occluded, the ischemic line could be the guidance for the parenchyma dissection (Figs. 9.3 and 9.4).

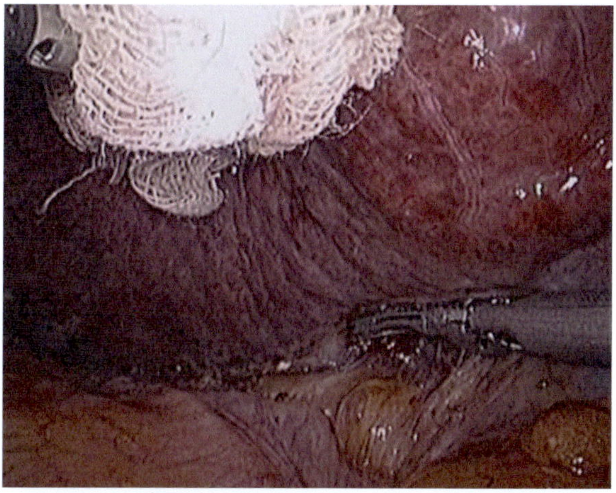

Fig. 9.2 The transection of the ligament of left vena cava

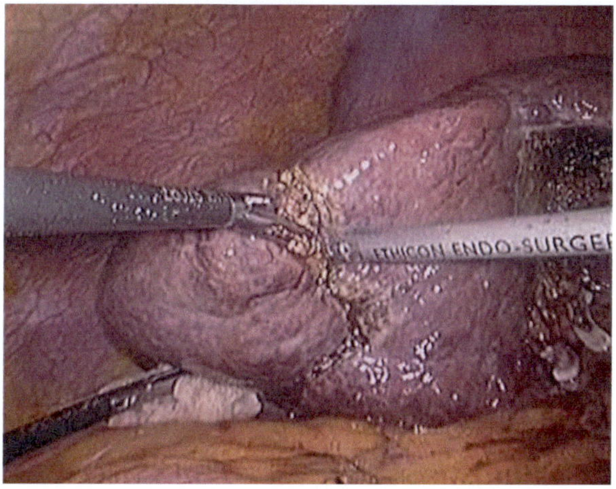

Fig. 9.3 Dissection of the superficial parenchyma of the right posterior section with harmonic scalpel

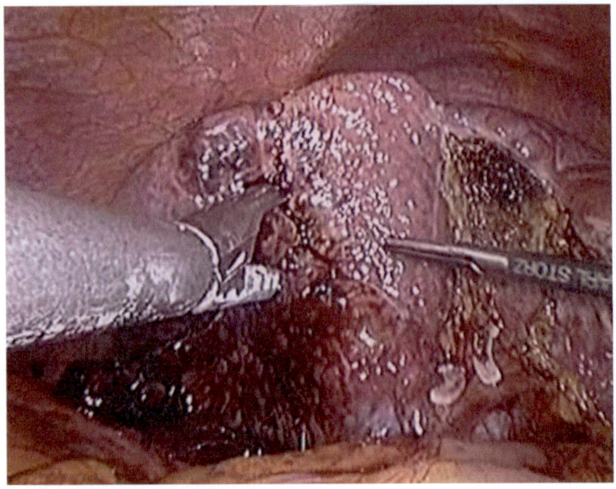

Fig. 9.4 Transection of the right posterior portal pedicels

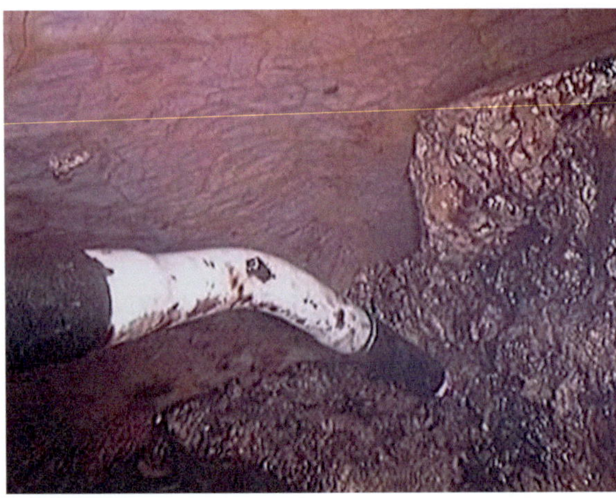

Fig. 9.5 Hemostasis in the raw surface

9.2.5 Control of Outflow Blood

There is no need for isolation of the hepatic vein of the right posterior section before the parenchyma dissection. For those with great risk of intraoperative bleeding, the second hilum should be clearly dissected without ligation. The hepatic vein of the right posterior section could be transected along with the parenchyma or clipped individually.

9.2.6 Hemostasis

The argon beam is used for errhysis of the raw surface (Fig. 9.5). The Biclamp is used for gentle active bleeding. The absorbable clips are used for obvious active bleeding. The suture is used for bile leak and the bleeding impossible to be controlled by other means.

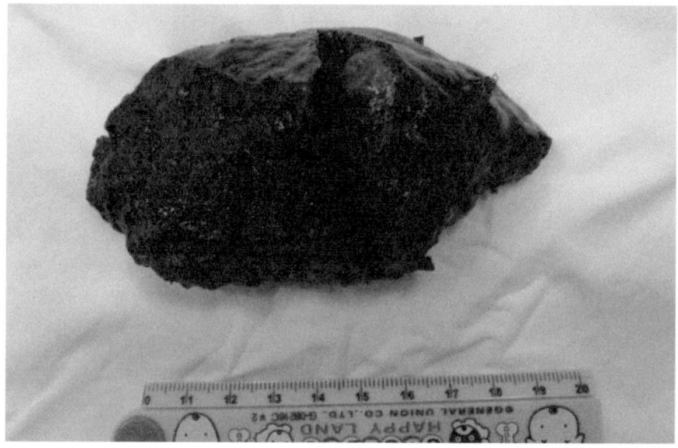

Fig. 9.6 The specimen

9.2.7 To Withdraw Specimen

The specimen is withdrawn with an endoscopic retriever through the expanded incision. It should be inspected immediately (Fig. 9.6).

9.2.8 Drainage

The two drainage tubes are placed on the raw surface of the liver and the foramen of Winslow, respectively.

9.3 Key Techniques

1. Bleeding. The first hilum should be well prepared in case of the need for Pringle maneuver. The timely conversion is a wise surgical strategy.
2. Bile leak. The absorbable clip or Hom-o-Lok should be used before transection of the bile ducts on the raw surface.

9.4 Complications

The intraoperative and postoperative complications can be managed similarly to those of laparoscopic lateral sectionectomy. Also see discussion in Chap. 1.

9.5 Notes

The gastrointestinal decompression and ureteral catheterization can stop on the first postoperative day. The patient can intake liquid diet. After 3–5 days, the patient can be discharged.

Retroperitoneal Laparoscopic Hepatectomy

10

Abstract

As a novel operation, retroperitoneal laparoscopic hepatectomy was conducted first by Dr. Liu Rong (Hu et al. 2011). It is a new option of liver minimal invasive surgeries.

As a novel operation, retroperitoneal laparoscopic hepatectomy was conducted first by Dr. Liu Rong (Hu et al. 2011). It is a new option of liver minimal invasive surgeries.

10.1 Indications

The right posterior section of the liver is closely adhesive to the posterior abdominal wall, with an adjacent relationship with the kidney, right adrenal gland, and IVC. The dissection in this potential plane can damage the hepatic short vein and parenchyma, causing bleeding. Enlightened by urological surgery, the access could directly reach the right back of the liver retroperitoneally. The primary clinical practices have showed that it is safe and feasible and also expands the indications of laparoscopic hepatectomy to some extent.

However, the indications for retroperitoneal laparoscopic hepatectomy are quite narrow: the superficial tumor located in the right posterior section with a diameter of $\leq$3 cm. Laparoscopic exploration of the abdominal cavity is impossible to perform with this approach. For those patients with severe abdominal adhesions, this approach may be a preferable alternative (Fig. 10.1).

R. Liu, *Laparoscopic Liver Resection*,
https://doi.org/10.1007/978-94-017-9735-1_10

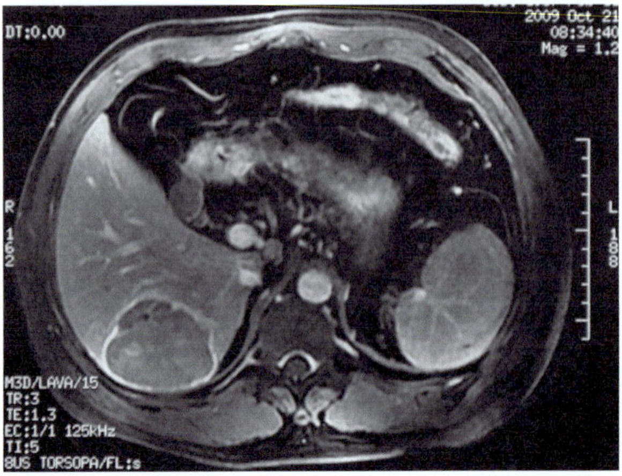

Fig. 10.1 Indications for the retroperitoneal laparoscopic hepatectomy

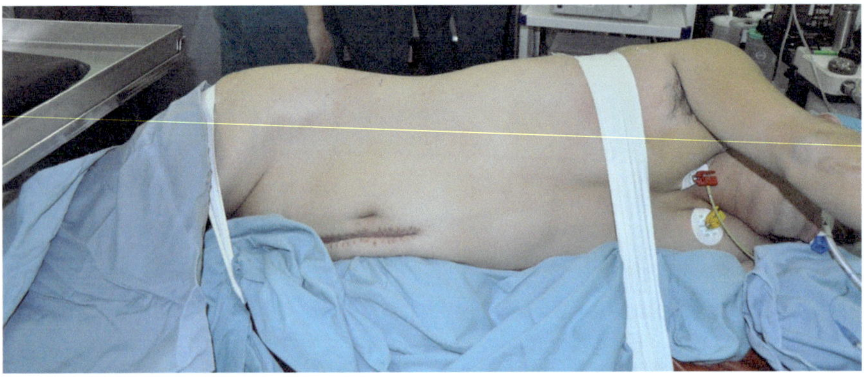

Fig. 10.2 Position of the patient (anterior)

10.2 Steps

The patient is in the left lateral recumbent position (Figs. 10.2 and 10.3). The pneumoperitoneum pressure is set at 14 mmHg.

The first trocar (10 mm) is placed using the same method as that of retroperitoneal laparoscopic adrenalectomy. Three additional trocars are then placed at 10 mm above the iliac crest in the midaxillary line (observation port), at 12 mm below the costal margin of the 11th rib on the anterior axillary line, and at 5 mm below the costal margin of the 12th rib on the posterior axillary line, respectively.

After the retroperitoneal space is established, the retroperitoneal fat tissue is dissociated from top to bottom. The lateroconal fascia and perinephric fascias are exposed. The perinephric space is opened by dissection of the lateroconal fascia and perinephric fascias at the peritoneal reflection. The perirenal fat capsule is divided along the prerenal fascia and then the perinephric space is expanded (Fig. 10.4).

The liver lies on the top of the perinephric space and anterior to the right adrenal gland (Fig. 10.5). The segment 6 can be exposed once the peritoneum is dissected. The tumor is removed by harmonica scalpel (Figs. 10.6 and 10.7).

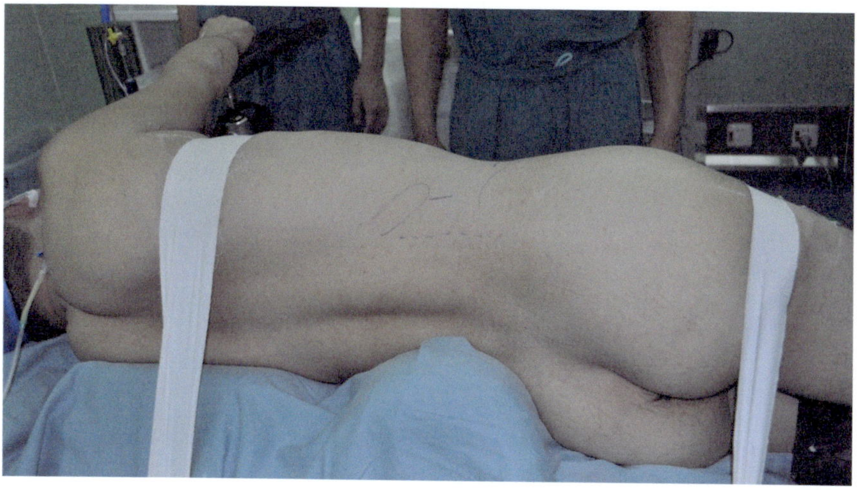

Fig. 10.3 Position of the patient (posterior)

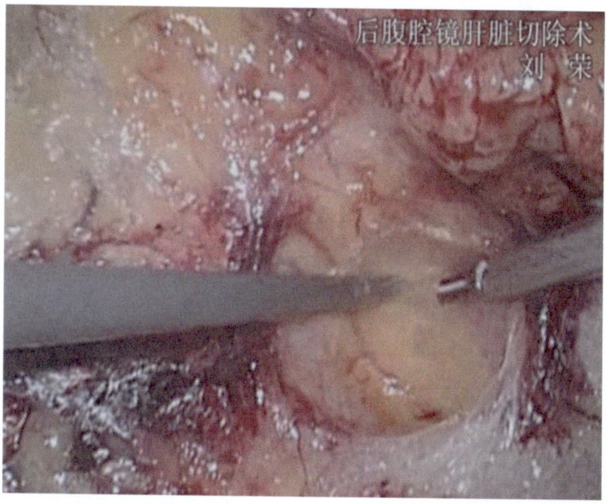

Fig. 10.4 Dissection of the perirenal fat

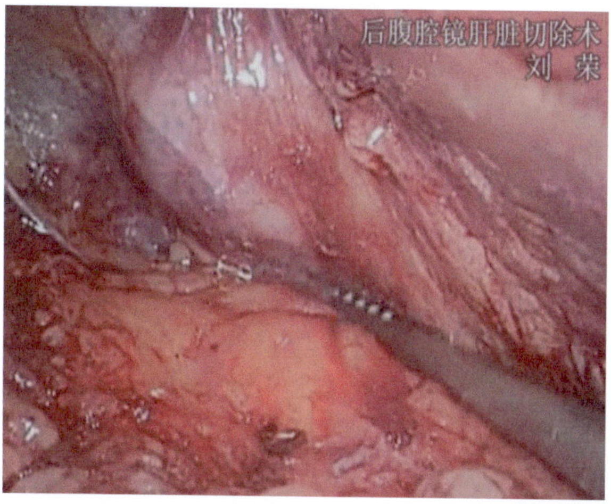

Fig. 10.5 The liver lies on the top of the perinephric space

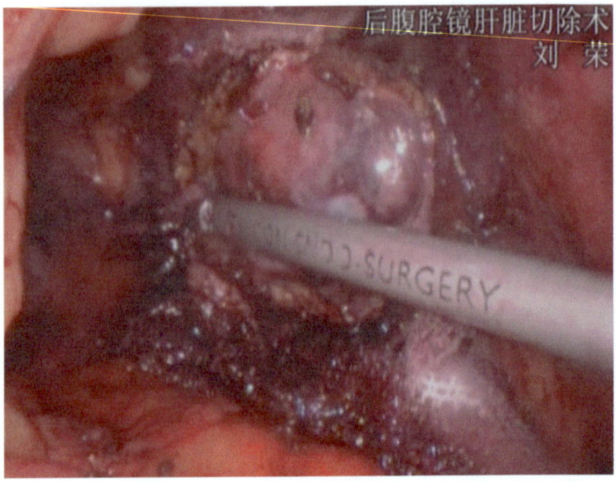

Fig. 10.6 The tumor is removed by harmonica scalpel

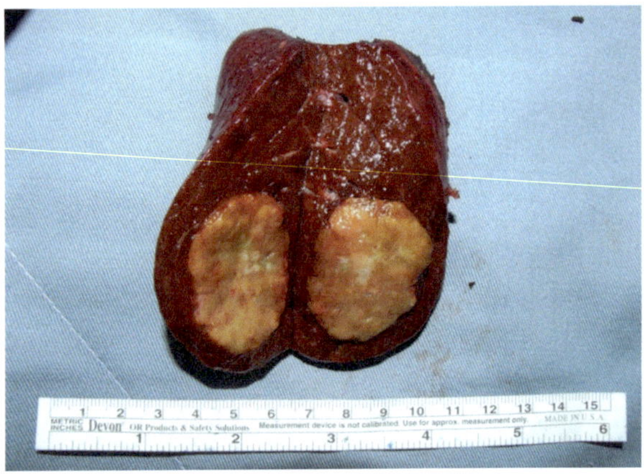

Fig. 10.7 The specimen

Reference

Hu M, et al. Retroperitoneal laparoscopic hepatectomy: a novel approach. Surg Laparosc Endosc Percutan Tech. 2011;21(5):e245–8.

11 Laparoscopic Right Hepatectomy

Abstract
Although the laparoscopic left lateral liver resection has been deemed as a gold standard procedure for liver lesions located in segments II and III, totally laparoscopic hemihepatectomy, especially laparoscopic right hepatectomy (LRH) is still a challenging and technically demanding surgery, with a high rate of conversion. There is general agreement that this surgery should be performed only at specialized centers with extensive experience in hepatic surgery and advanced laparoscopic technique, to ensure patients' safety and strict adherence to established surgical indications. Our team has experience in performing laparoscopic hepatectomy for over 10 years. After establishing stylized method for laparoscopic right hemihepatectomy (LRH), we had accomplished 21 totally laparoscopic right hepatectomy from 2011 to 2014. In this chapter, we describe our technique for stylized method of laparoscopic right hepatectomy, highlighting the most relevant technical details essential for accomplishing a safe and efficient procedure. We also discuss the indications of increasing experience and improved skills developing during this time.

Although the laparoscopic left lateral liver resection has been deemed as a gold standard procedure for liver lesions located in segments II and III, totally laparoscopic hemihepatectomy, especially laparoscopic right hepatectomy (LRH) is still a challenging and technically demanding surgery, with a high rate of conversion. There is general agreement that this surgery should be performed only at specialized centers with extensive experience in hepatic surgery and advanced laparoscopic technique, to ensure patients' safety and strict adherence to established surgical indications. Our team has experience in performing laparoscopic hepatectomy for over 10 years. After establishing stylized method for laparoscopic right hemihepatectomy (LRH), we had accomplished 21 totally laparoscopic right

R. Liu, *Laparoscopic Liver Resection*,
https://doi.org/10.1007/978-94-017-9735-1_11

hepatectomy from 2011 to 2014. In this chapter, we describe our technique for stylized method of laparoscopic right hepatectomy, highlighting the most relevant technical details essential for accomplishing a safe and efficient procedure. We also discuss the indications of increasing experience and improved skills developing during this time.

11.1 Indications and Contraindications

Patients' general conditions should not compromise the safety of the anesthesia, and ASA classification (American Society of Anesthesiologists' Physical Status Classification) should be at 3 or below. The preoperative investigations of lesion included liver imaging (spiral computed tomography or magnetic resonance imaging). For patients with cirrhosis undergoing major hepatectomy, Child-Pugh classification, the ICG (indocyanine green) clearance test, and computed tomography volumetry are helpful in evaluating whether the remnant liver volume is adequate.

The indications for LRH are similar to those for open liver resection with the same oncologic rules, including "no-touch" tumor technique, radical R0 resection, and a free surgical margin. Benign or malignant lesions located in the right lobe of the liver, involving the Segment 5–8 or adjacent to main inflow/outflow vessels of the right lobe of liver are considered suitable for right hepatectomy.

The need for vascular or biliary reconstruction is currently a contraindication to the laparoscopic approach. Preoperative imaging or intraoperative ultrasonography that fails to delineate the location of the lesion clearly or could not obtain a negative resection margin should be considered a relative contraindication. Previous abdominal surgery history increases the likelihood of conversion, but is not a contraindication to the minimally invasive approach.

11.2 Procedure

11.2.1 Patient's Position and Trocar Arrangement

Under general anesthesia, the patient is placed in left lateral semi-decubitus position with the right arm suspended. A Veress needle is inserted 5 cm right of the midline at the level of the umbilicus and the peritoneal cavity is insufflated to a pneumoperitoneum with a pressure of 15 mmHg and the Veress needle is withdrawn. The laparoscopic camera is inserted through the trocar at the puncture point of Veress needle. Three or four working trocars are placed along the line just beneath the costal arch. One of them is the 12-mm key working trocar, which would be used to handle the endostapler, and the other assistant trocars are placed at intervals of 8–10 cm next to that. Selection of every point to insert trocar should depend on the liver's shape, key anatomy structure, and decreasing the mutual interference of the instruments during the operation.

11.2.2 Laparoscopic Ultrasonography

We use the Pro Focus 2202 Ultrasound Scanner system with Laparoscopic Transducer (Fig. 11.1). The procedure of intraoperative ultrasound (IOUS) is as follows: (1) Screen the entire liver to rule out any satellite nodule of HCC; (2) Identify surgical resection margin; (3) Assess the anatomical structures such as vascular and biliary branches in order to accomplish anatomical resections.

11.2.3 Mobilization of the Right Lobe

We first divide the round and falciform ligaments to the level of the second porta hepatis (Fig. 11.2). Then completely divide the right triangular and coronary ligaments, and the bare area of the right lobe is mobilized completely (Fig. 11.3). The inferior vena cava is dissected and small accessory hepatic veins can be controlled with Hem-o-lok surgical clips (Fig. 11.4). The right hepatic vein (RHV) is exposed and the retrocaval ligament is divided to allow access to the right side of the vein, when the right hepatic vein cannot be dissected safely from an extrahepatic approach, this dissection should be completed within the liver parenchyma.

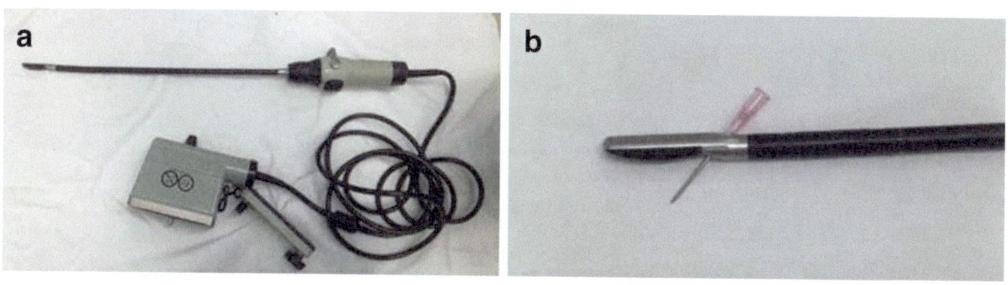

Fig. 11.1 The laparoscopic ultrasound transducer. (**a**) the general view of the transducer; (**b**) the guiding tunnel of the transducer

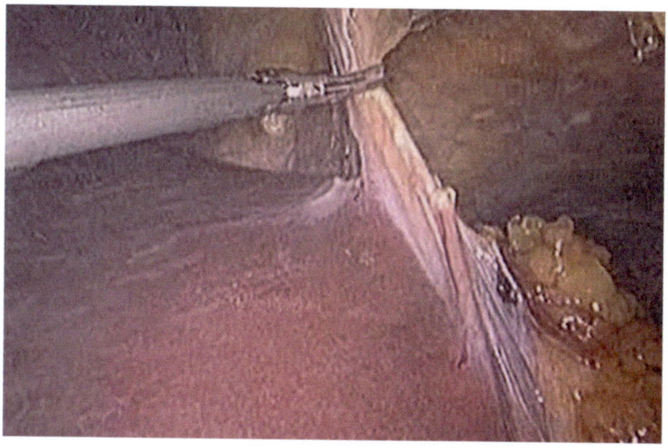

Fig. 11.2 Dissection of the round and falciform ligaments

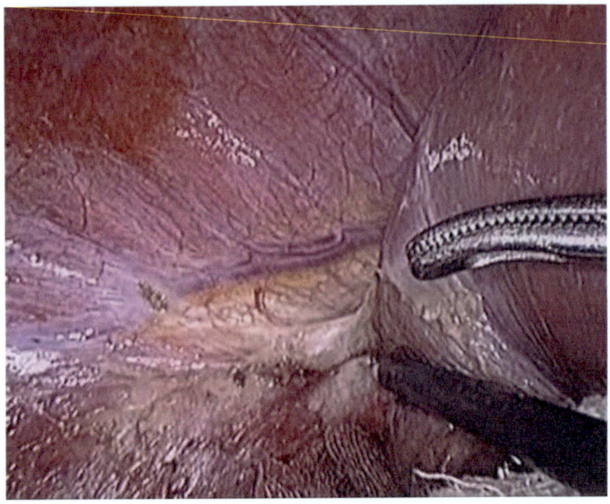

Fig. 11.3 Dissection of the right triangular and coronary ligaments

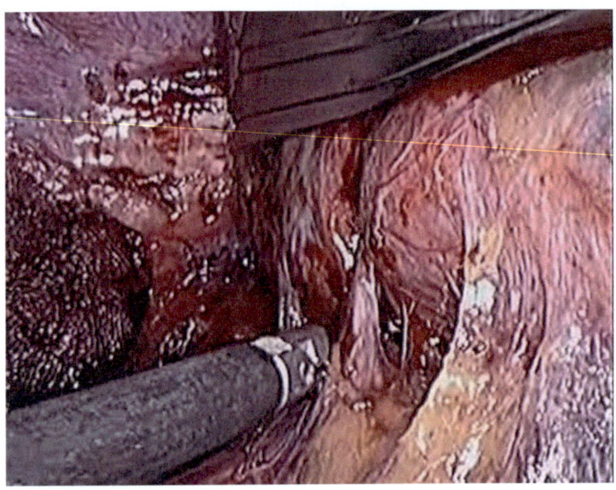

Fig. 11.4 Dissection of small accessory hepatic veins

11.2.4 Control of the Inflow/Outflow Vessels

After cholecystectomy, hilar dissection is performed to free the right Glisson's pedicle. Firstly, the right hepatic artery is identified, ligated, and transected (Fig. 11.5). Secondly, the portal vein is traced until the bifurcating into its right or left branch, then the right branch of portal vein is ligated but not transected to obstruction inflow (Fig. 11.6). CT angiography is a useful way to evaluate the variation of right portal vein before the operation.

Normally, we should not attempt to dissect and expose the right hepatic vein extraparenchymally, because handling the bleeding of RHV laparoscopically is very difficult and has the potential risk of gas embolism (Fig. 11.7). If there are no thick

Fig. 11.5 (**a, b**) Ligation and transection of the right hepatic artery

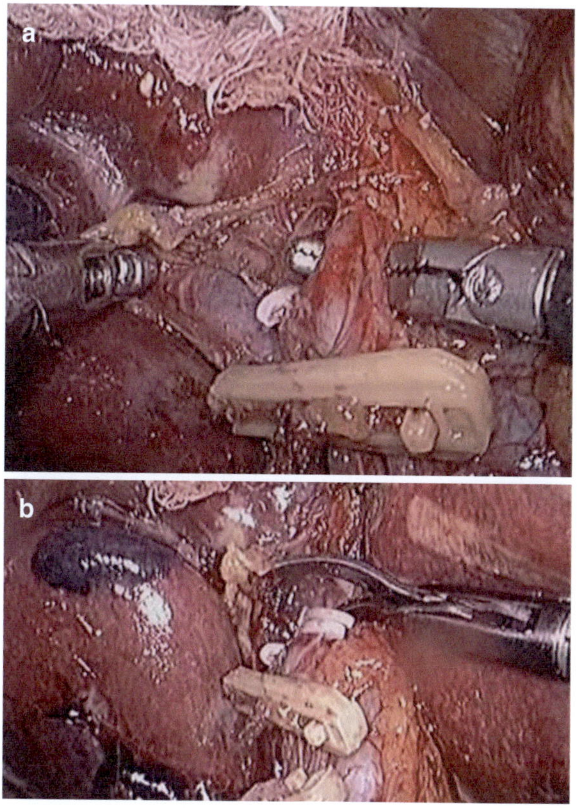

tributaries near the root of RHV and the surrounding tissue of the RHV could be identified and dissected free easily, the root of the RHV is fully exposed from the anterocranial and the posterior aspects by dividing the right retrocaval ligament. The RHV itself is transected with endostapler until the accomplishment of the parenchymal division. Experienced surgeon could divide RHV and hang it with silicon tube or a cotton tape that could control the massive bleeding of the RHV during the transection of the hepatic parenchyma.

11.2.5 Transection of the Hepatic Parenchyma

The superficial hepatic parenchyma is transected using the Harmonic Scalpel (Ethicon, Cincinnati, OH, USA) or the THUNDERBEAT (Olympus, Tokyo, Japan) (Figs. 11.8 and 11.9), the deeper portion of the parenchyma is dissected combined with the BiClamp® forceps of Electronic Surgical Workstation and Argon beam coagulation to achieve venous hemostasis (Fig. 11.10). Bipolar coagulating/cutting

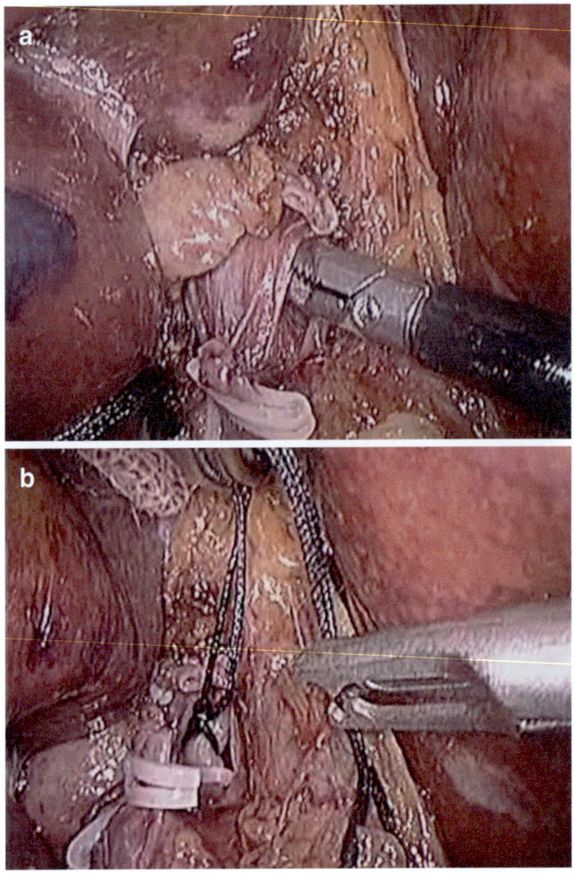

Fig. 11.6 (**a, b**) Ligation and transection of the right branch of portal vein

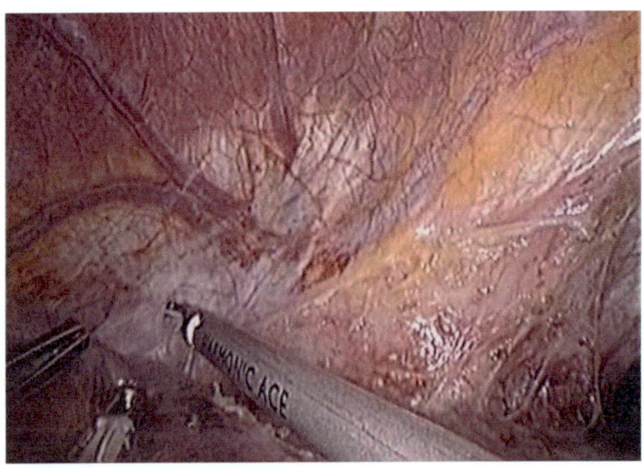

Fig. 11.7 Dissection and exposion of the RHV

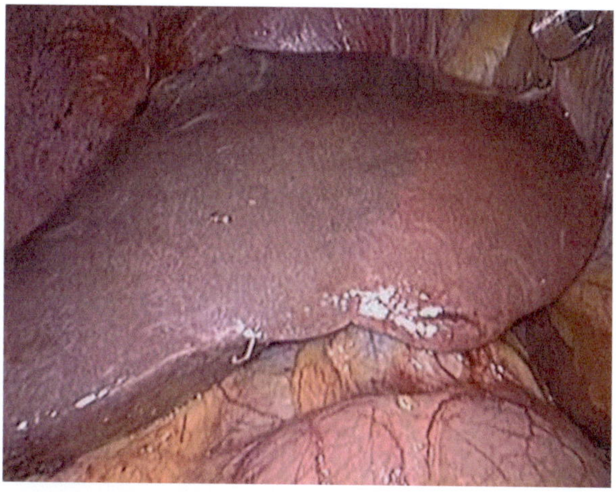

Fig. 11.8 The ischemic line of the liver surface

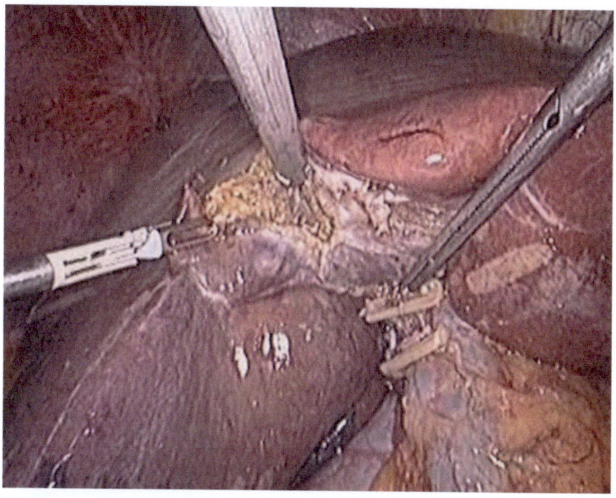

Fig. 11.9 Transection of superficial hepatic parenchyma

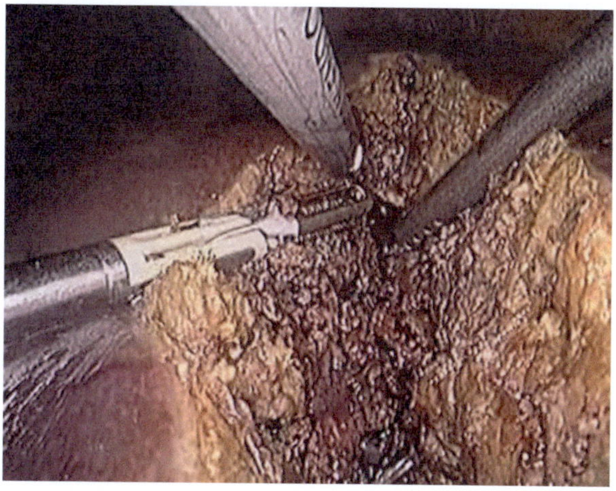

Fig. 11.10 Transection and hemostasis of the deeper portion of the parenchyma

device (LigaSure, Valley Laboratory, Boulder, CO) is an instrument of choice to seal vessels that are less than 7 mm (e.g., small venous branches or glissonian pedicle). The plane of dissection should be slightly "open" faced to camera by the assistant to obtaining good views. Laparoscopic cavitron ultrasonic dissector can be used to transect the parenchyma also. Lapro-Clip™ absorbable clip or Hem-o-lok is used to transect vessels and bile ducts up to 12 mm (Fig. 11.11). Endoscopic articulating linear cutter (such as Echelon, Ethicon, Endo-Surgery) facilitates division of larger vessels (right hepatic vein or right hepatic pedicle) (Figs. 11.12 and 11.13).

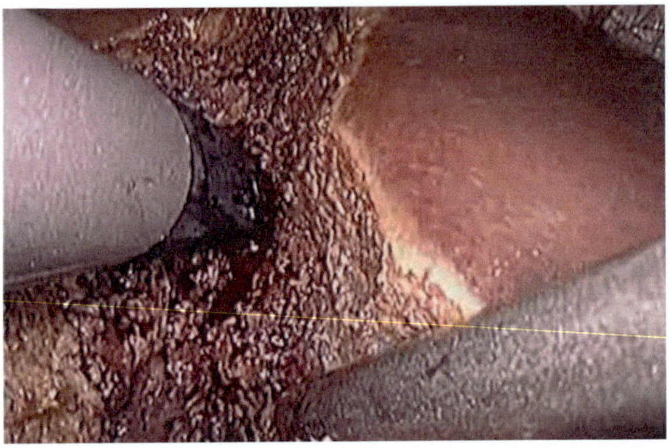

Fig. 11.11 The absorbable chip for the vessels in raw surface

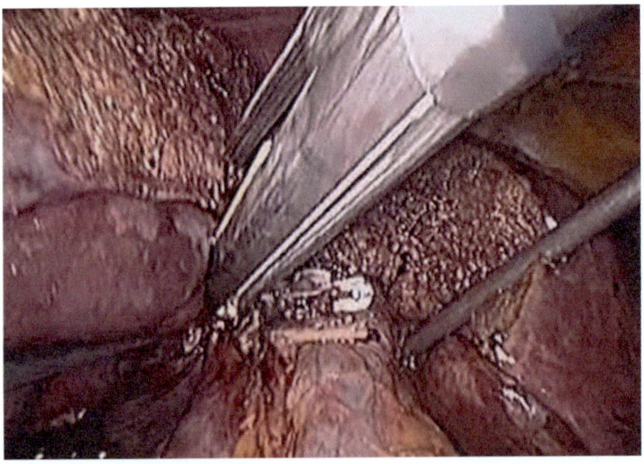

Fig. 11.12 Transection of the right portal pedicels

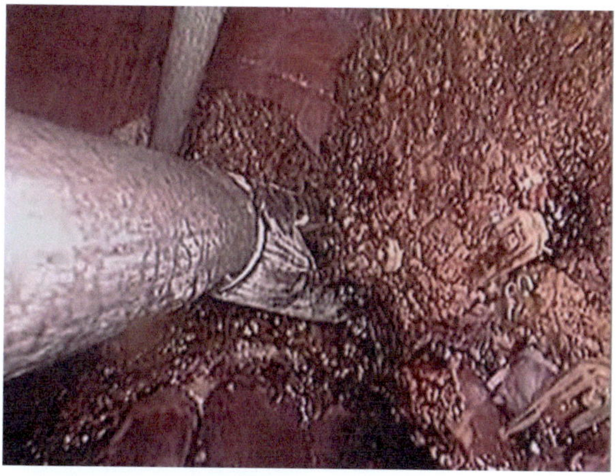

Fig. 11.13 Transection of the right hepatic vein

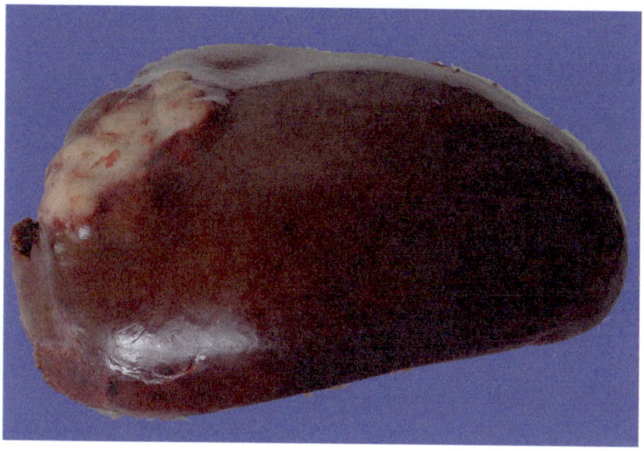

Fig. 11.14 The specimen

11.2.6 Specimen Retrieval and Drainage

The specimen is removed in a plastic bag (Endocatch; Ethicon Endo-Surgery) introduced through one of 12-mm ports which is subsequently extended to a 7–10 cm incision.

After retrieving the specimen (Fig. 11.14), the raw surface of the liver is examined carefully for bleeding and bile leak. Hemostasis is obtained using BiClamp® forceps of Electronic Surgical Workstation and Argon beam coagulation (Fig. 11.15). Bile leak is controlled with Prolene 4/0 stitches or with clips. A 20Fr silicon tube drain is positioned near the resection surface.

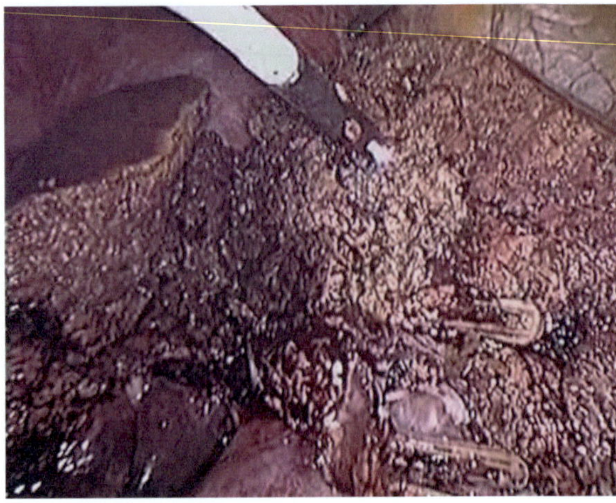

Fig. 11.15 Hemostasis in the raw surface by Argon beam coagulation

11.3 Key Techniques

Left lateral semi-decubitus position with the right arm suspended has several privileges for the hepatectomy: Firstly, with this position surgeon could view the hilum from the right posterior side that makes the hilar dissection more accurate. Secondly, the weight of the liver makes the right lobe naturally falls to the left, which helps to dissect the coronary and right triangular ligaments. Thirdly, transection plane could be easily kept to face the camera.

The ultrasonic dissector is mainly applied to perform tissue dissection and hemostasis while the BiClamp® forceps in the left hand provide retraction and rescue hemostasis. BiClamp® forceps have been very useful for hemostasis and coagulation of liver parenchyma and small vessels (<4 mm). The assistant should keep the surgical field clean and visualize the bleeding point with suction. The transection of parenchyma should be advanced layer after layer. That is important to avoid tunneling into the hepatic parenchyma accidently, thus creating deep holes where the view is compromised and bleeding control is difficult. The active blade of ultrasonic shears have a potential risk of massive bleeding by direct injury of the wall of hepatic veins, so that it is better to avoid exposure of the major trunk of middle hepatic vein on the transection plane. Accurate anatomic selection of transection plane requires the help of ultrasonography. Bleeding from injury on the venous wall can usually be managed by direct compression with gauze pad and "close" the transection surface and be careful not to coagulate blindly. Major injury of hepatic vein trunk should be sutured and stumps of thick tributaries should be clipped. Recent studies suggest that critical gas embolism is unlikely to occur as long as the liver parenchyma is dissected under carbon dioxide insufflation at pressure below 12 mmHg.

11.4 Complications

Bleeding is always the most important issue in laparoscopic hepatectomy and it is the most frequent reason that causes fear among surgeons. Thus, surgeons who perform laparoscopic right hepatic resection should be familiar with the laparoscopic anatomy of the liver and laparoscopic suturing. After retrieving the specimen, the raw surface of liver should be examined carefully for bleeding and bile leak. Laparotomy is the ultimate and most effective way to control the bleeding.

Symptomatic pleural effusion could be managed conservatively without the need for additional surgery.

11.5 Notes

Be careful of the volume and characteristics of drainage fluid. The gastrointestinal decompression can stop after 6–8 hours and the patient can intake liquid diet.

Laparoscopic Caudate Lobectomy

12

Abstract

Caudate lobe is surrounded by most major vessels of the liver, which makes laparoscopic hepatectomy of caudate lobe more complex and potentially more dangerous than other hepatic segmentectomy. Such dangerous procedures should be performed by surgeons who have advanced experiences both in open and minimally invasive liver resection. The caudate lobe is the dorsal portion of the liver and half encircles the IVC, and it is composed of three parts: Spiegel lobe lies to the left side of IVC; the paracaval portion lies anterior to the IVC, and the caudate process is located between the posterior branch of the right Glissonian and IVC. Safe laparoscopic resection of caudate lobe requires mobilization and control of the inflow/outflow vessels of the caudate lobe.

Caudate lobe is surrounded by most major vessels of the liver, which makes laparoscopic hepatectomy of caudate lobe more complex and potentially more dangerous than other hepatic segmentectomy. Such dangerous procedures should be performed by surgeons who have advanced experiences both in open and minimally invasive liver resection. The caudate lobe is the dorsal portion of the liver and half encircles the IVC, and it is composed of three parts: Spiegel lobe lies to the left side of IVC; the paracaval portion lies anterior to the IVC, and the caudate process is located between the posterior branch of the right Glissonian and IVC. Safe laparoscopic resection of caudate lobe requires mobilization and control of the inflow/outflow vessels of the caudate lobe.

R. Liu, *Laparoscopic Liver Resection*,
https://doi.org/10.1007/978-94-017-9735-1_12

12.1 Indications and Contraindications

Symptomatic benign tumors or malignant tumors in the caudate lobe are indications for laparoscopic caudate lobectomy. For the anatomical features of caudate lobe, the lesions that are amenable for laparoscopic resection are mostly located in the Spiegel lobe and caudate process.

Contraindications for laparoscopic caudate resection include portal vein/IVC invasion, large tumor volume, and insufficient experience of the surgeon.

12.2 Procedure

12.2.1 Laparoscopic Hepatectomy of Spiegel Lobe

12.2.1.1 Patient's Position and Trocar Arrangement

Under general anesthesia, the patient is placed in supine position. A Veress needle is inserted below the umbilicus. Then the peritoneal cavity is insufflated to a pneumoperitoneum with a pressure of 13 mmHg and the Veress needle is withdrawn. A trocar for the laparoscopic camera is inserted through the same incision. Three or four working trocars are placed along the line just beneath the costal arch. One of them is the 12-mm key working trocar, which would be used to handle the endostapler, and the other assist trocars are placed at intervals of 8–10 cm next to that. The trocar arrangement should depend on the liver's shape and key anatomy structure, while decreasing the mutual interference of the instruments during the operation.

12.2.1.2 Mobilization

We first divide the round ligament and take down the falciform ligaments from the abdominal wall to the confluence of the hepatic veins and vena cava. The round ligament should be transected close to the abdominal wall as to avoid interfering the view by its dangling remnant. Then the left triangular and coronary ligaments are divided completely (Fig. 12.1), and subsequently the assistant can retract the left lateral lobe and divided the lesser omentum, so that the speigel lobe can be exposed (Fig. 12.2). IVC is dissected and small accessory hepatic veins can be controlled with Hem-o-lok surgical clips (Fig. 12.3). During the whole period of operation, surgeon should be very careful of these clips and fall off any one of them may cause bleeding. When the left hepatocaval ligament is divided and the Spiegel lobe mobilized away from IVC, the root of LHV is exposed (Fig. 12.4).

Hilar dissection is performed to free the left Glisson's pedicle. The caudate branches of the left portal vein and hepatic artery are dissected and transection by the Hem-o-lok or absorbable clip (Fig. 12.5).

12.2.1.3 Transection of the Hepatic Parenchyma

The isthmus of the caudate lobe is transected using the Harmonic Scalpel combined with the bipolar forceps (Fig. 12.6). Then absorbable clip or endoscopic articulating linear cutter is used to transect the parenchyma depending on the thickness of isthmus. It should be very careful to avoid the injury of HV/IVC by the tip of linear cutter.

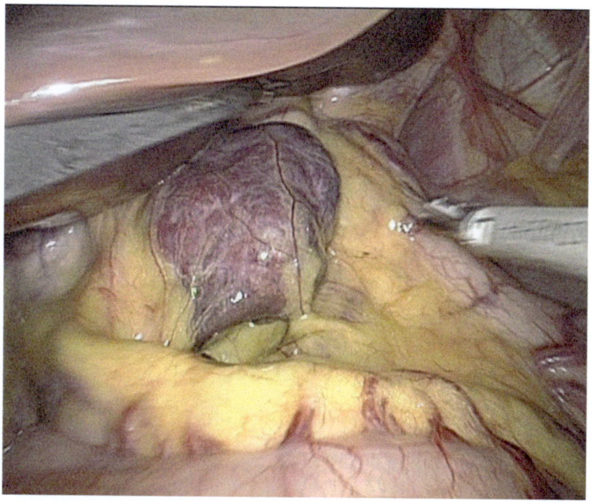

Fig. 12.1 Mobilization the left triangular and coronary ligaments

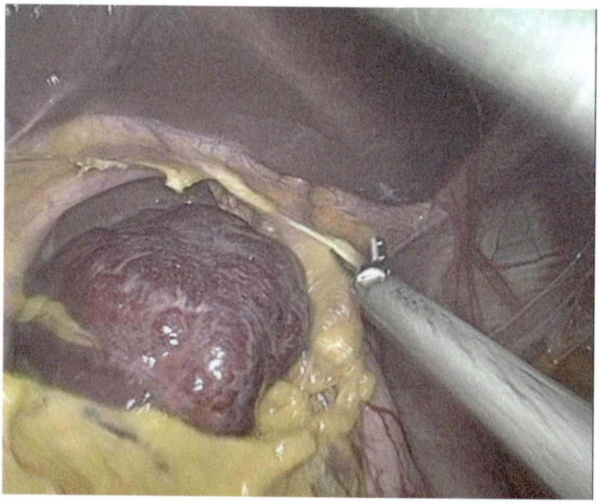

Fig. 12.2 Exposure of the speigel lobe

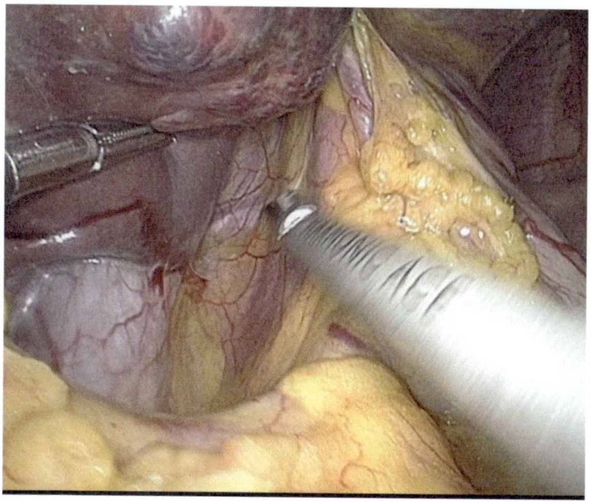

Fig. 12.3 Dissection of the IVC

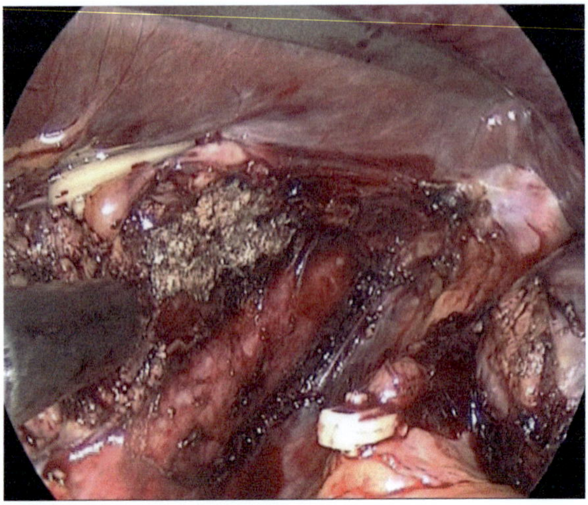

Fig. 12.4 Exposure of the root of LHV

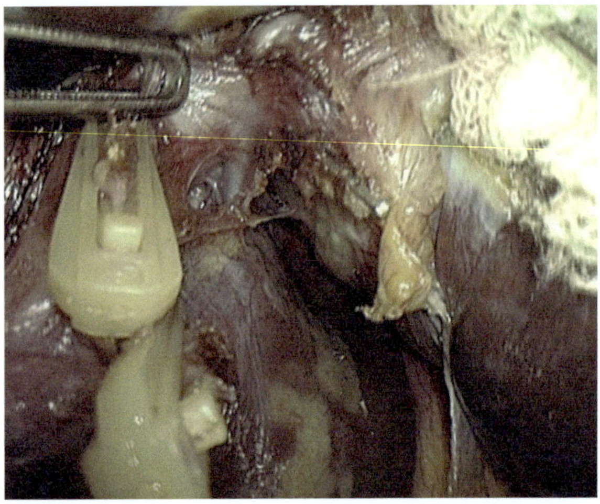

Fig. 12.5 Dissection of the caudate branches of the left portal vein

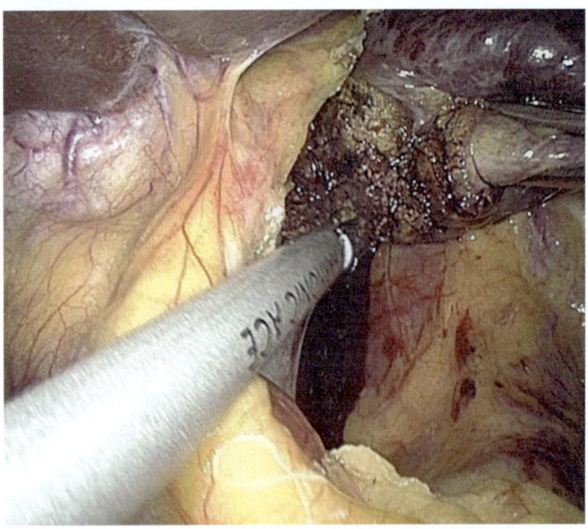

Fig. 12.6 Transection of the hepatic parenchyma

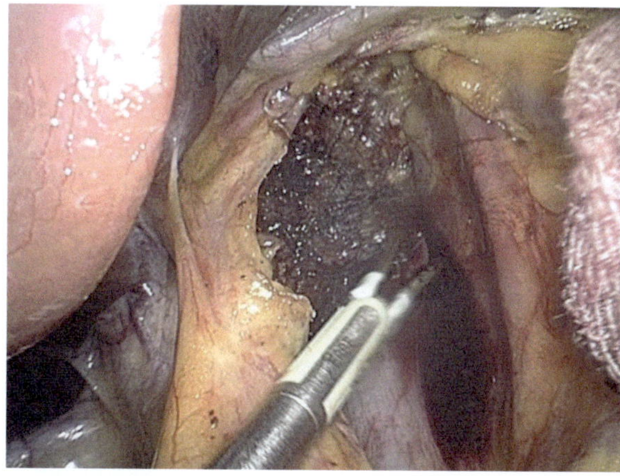

Fig. 12.7 Hemostasis in the raw surface

12.2.1.4 Specimen Retrieval and Drainage

The specimen is removed in a plastic bag (Endocatch; Ethicon Endo-Surgery) introduced through one of 12-mm ports subsequently extended to a 7–10 cm incision.

After retrieving the specimen, the raw surface of the liver is examined carefully for bleeding and bile leak. Hemostasis is obtained using BiClamp® forceps of Electronic Surgical Workstation and Argon beam coagulation (Fig. 12.7). Bile leak is controlled with Prolene 4/0 stitches or with clips. A 20Fr silicon tube drain is positioned near the resection surface.

12.2.2 Laparoscopic Hepatectomy of Caudate Process

Only specific lesions in the caudate process are amenable to laparoscopic resection. We have performed the laparoscopic hepatectomy of the caudate process as follows:

12.2.2.1 Patient's Position and Trocar Arrangement

The patient is placed in the supine position. Arrangements of trocar are same with that of the laparoscopic right hepatectomy, and three working trocars were placed along the line just beneath the costal arch.

12.2.2.2 Mobilization

We first divide the small accessory hepatic veins and mobilized the lesion. The small hepatic veins can be controlled with Hem-o-lok surgical clips or absorbable clips.

12.2.2.3 Transection of the Hepatic Parenchyma

The parenchyma is transected using the Harmonic Scalpel combined with the bipolar forceps. Then absorbable clips are used to control the vessels of lesion.

12.2.2.4 Specimen Retrieval and Drainage

The specimen is removed in a plastic bag (Endocatch; Ethicon Endo-Surgery) introduced through one of 12-mm ports.

After retrieving the specimen, the raw surface of liver is examined carefully for bleeding. Hemostasis is obtained using BiClamp® forceps or Argon beam coagulation.

12.3 Key Techniques

Mobilization is the key step for the laparoscopic caudate lobectomy, and surgeon should have enough experience in handing the small hepatic vein.

12.4 Complications

IVC/HV bleeding is the most dangerous issue in laparoscopic hepatectomy of caudate lobe and has potential risk of gas embolism. Thus, surgeons who perform laparoscopic hepatic caudate lobe resection should be familiar with the laparoscopic anatomy of the liver and laparoscopic suturing. If the bleeding is difficult to handle, surgeon should take temporary measures for bleeding control if possible, and the conversion to laparotomy must be performed without hesitation.

12.5 Notes

Pay attention to observe the drainage fluid and in case of hemorrhage or bile leakage.

Radiofrequency Ablation Assisted Laparoscopic Hepatectomy

13

Abstract

As is introduced in the above chapters, despite advances in surgical technique, due to poor hepatic reserve, portal hypertension and other conditions that patients with concomitant cirrhosis may have, laparoscopic liver resection may be encountered with considerable intraoperative blood loss, which is why it is essential to develop techniques that can reduce blood loss during liver parenchymal resection. Radiofrequency ablation (RFA), which had been proved to be able to block small and medium-sized blood vessels (less than 5 mm in diameter) in the liver through thermal coagulation, was used in liver resection to reduce bleeding in the past years with satisfying results (Weber et al. 2002; Pai et al. 2008), and thus has been recommended for cirrhotic patients. In this chapter, we will discuss the indications and contraindications, operative steps, key techniques, major complications as well as points should be noted of RFA assisted laparoscopic liver resection in this chapter.

As is introduced in the above chapters, despite advances in surgical technique, due to poor hepatic reserve, portal hypertension and other conditions that patients with concomitant cirrhosis may have, laparoscopic liver resection may be encountered with considerable intraoperative blood loss, which is why it is essential to develop techniques that can reduce blood loss during liver parenchymal resection. Radiofrequency ablation (RFA), which had been proved to be able to block small and medium-sized blood vessels (less than 5 mm in diameter) in the liver through thermal coagulation, was used in liver resection to reduce bleeding in the past years with satisfying results (Weber et al. 2002; Pai et al. 2008), and thus has been recommended for cirrhotic patients. In this chapter, we will discuss the indications and contraindications, operative steps, key techniques, major complications as well as points should be noted of RFA assisted laparoscopic liver resection in this chapter.

R. Liu, *Laparoscopic Liver Resection*,
https://doi.org/10.1007/978-94-017-9735-1_13

13.1 Indications and Contraindications

The following inclusion criteria are recommended:

1. Resectable liver lesion or lesions with cirrhosis and adequate (R0) margins;
2. Hepatic function of Child-Pugh class A or B;
3. Adequate remaining functional liver parenchyma;
4. History of multiple TACE procedures.
5. Non-neoplastic lesions suitable for laparoscopic liver resection.

The following exclusion criteria were recommended:

1. History of abdominal surgery;
2. Uncontrollable ascites, hepatic encephalopathy, or variceal bleeding;
3. Dysfunction of other organs;
4. Extrahepatic spread of disease;
5. Extremely impaired liver function (Child-Pugh class C).

13.2 Steps

1. The key technical points of patient positioning, preoperative preparation, anesthesia, ports placement, and the exploration of tumors are similar for radiofrequency assisted laparoscopic liver resection with conventional laparoscopic liver resection, which has been introduced in detail in the above chapters. Laparoscopic ultrasonography should be performed to have a sufficient understanding of the number and location of the lesions, the detail of anatomical information of biliary and vascular structures, and also the direction of the puncture of the needle (Figs. 13.1, 13.2, and 13.3).

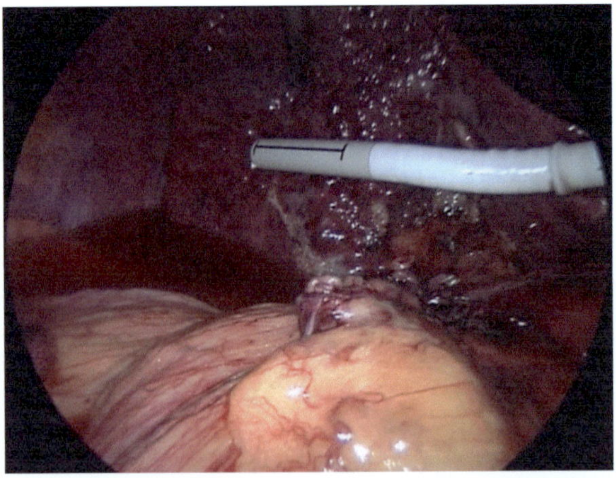

Fig. 13.1 Laparoscopic ultrasonography should be performed if necessary

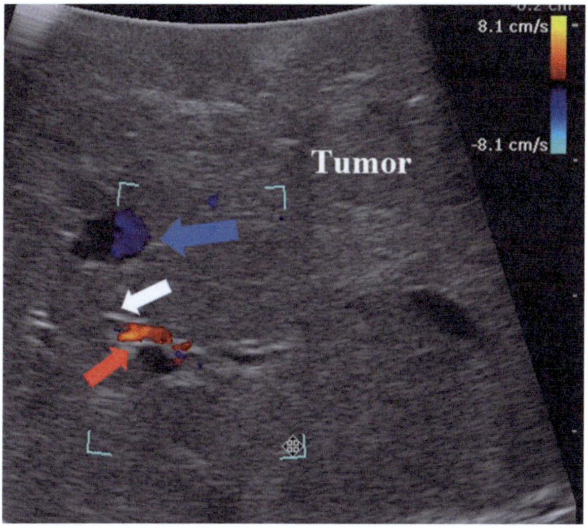

Fig. 13.2 Laparoscopic ultrasonography demonstrating the detailed anatomical information of biliary (*white arrow*) duct, hepatic artery (*red arrow*) and hepatic vascular (*blue arrow*)

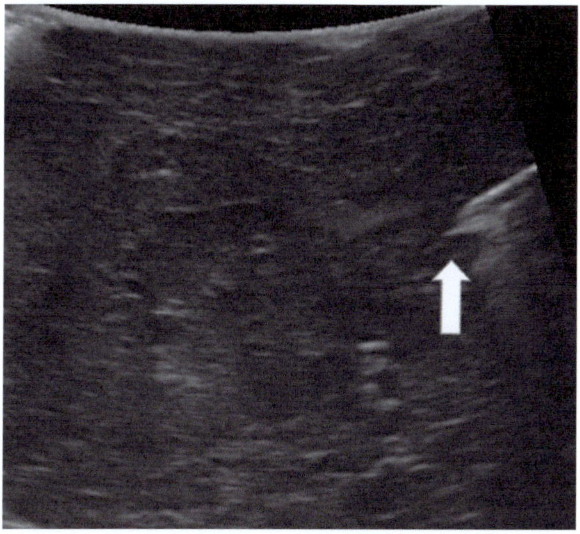

Fig. 13.3 Laparoscopic ultrasonography demonstrating the direction of needle (*arrow*)

2. After laparoscopic scanning of the liver, the surgical tumor resection margins can be demarcated. Generally, the margins should be kept 1 cm out the tumors, and RFA was performed using a 17-G cooled-tip electrode with a 2-cm metallic tip or 3-cm metallic tip (Figs. 13.4 and 13.5); the power was generally set to 60–80 W, and the coagulation time was usually 2–4 min. Bleeding vessels can be treated with an extra procedure in purpose if necessary (Fig. 13.6). The angle of

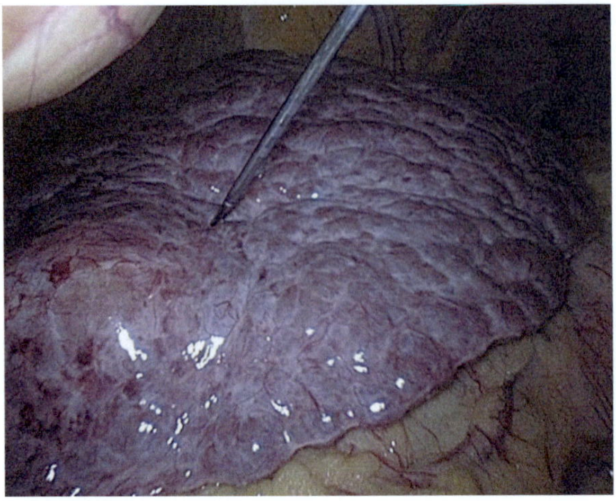

Fig. 13.4 The RFA needle

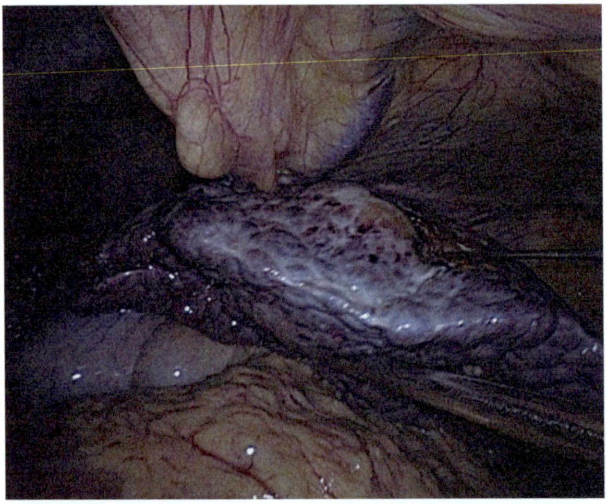

Fig. 13.5 The RFA is being performed before resection of hepatic tumor

the puncture of RF needle is extremely important, and generally should be kept similar with the following transection. After RFA, it can be hard to have a clear imaging of the tumor any more. Generally, RFA should be performed 2–3 cm each along the resection line, and sometimes a second application of RF ablation is necessary to achieve sufficient coagulation. For deep tumors, the RF ablation can be performed in the deepest part and then repeated after the needle tip is withdrawn to the superficial area. If large vessels are encountered, it is extremely important to reconsider the feasibility of the surgical plan. When the transection plane is close to a major vessel, the RF ablation should be performed closer to the vessel, with caution, in case the biliary structure or artery is injured.

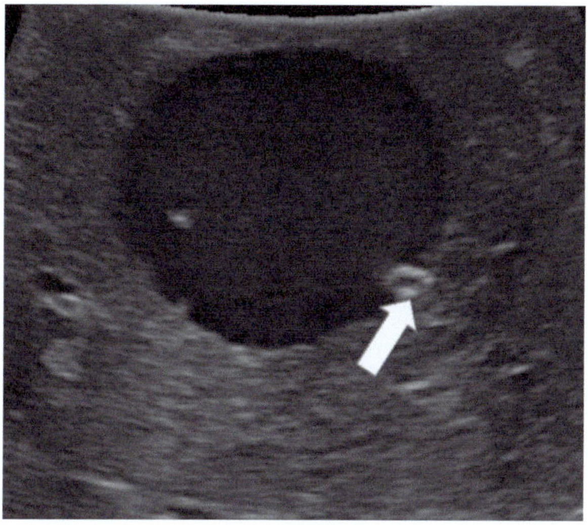

Fig. 13.6 A bleeding vessel of hepatic cellular carcinoma

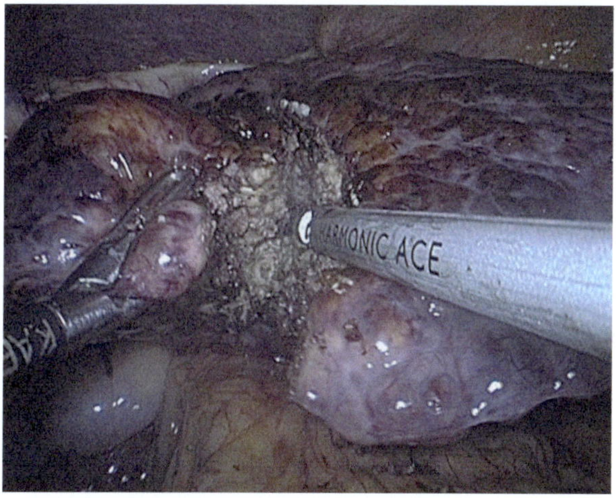

Fig. 13.7 Laparoscopic liver transection after RFA

3. Along the necrotic zone, laparoscopic liver transection can be achieved using an ultrasonic dissector or other energy devices (Fig. 13.7) and the resected specimen can be placed in a plastic bag and removed, which has been introduced in the previous chapters. During the operation, a formal hilar dissection and Pringle maneuver is generally unnecessary. Primary dissection or second hilar dissection was only done when the tumor was adjacent to the hepatic hilum or hepatic veins. With the assistance of radiofrequency ablation, the operative blood loss and transfusion rate can be minimized.

13.3 Key Techniques

1. A sufficient inspection using laparoscopic ultrasound to demarcate a rational and feasible transection plane is extremely important, which should take the remnant liver function, the encountered vessels, and the sufficiency of resection area into account. Generally, the angle of the puncture of RF needle should be kept parallel to the transection plane, which is why the puncture site should be carefully selected.
2. Laparoscopic ultrasound is routinely used to locate the tumors. Generally, hepatic cellular carcinoma appeared as hypo-echoic lesion (Fig. 13.8), and cirrhotic nodes appeared as hyper-echoic lesion with sharp margin which is usually smaller than 1 cm (Fig. 13.9). Sometimes malignant tumor might appear as inhomogeneous echoic lesion or iso-echoic lesion with no clear margin, in which case, contrast enhanced ultrasound is suggested for differential diagnosis (Figs. 13.10 and 13.11).
3. When the location of tumor is very deep, RFA might cause heat injury of the underneath structure such as the stomach and intestine. In this case, liver can be lifted or stuffed with gauze to protect the adjacent tissue.

13.4 Complications

The RF ablation assisted laparoscopic liver resection is generally safe and feasible, with very low complication rate. The major complications are as followed:

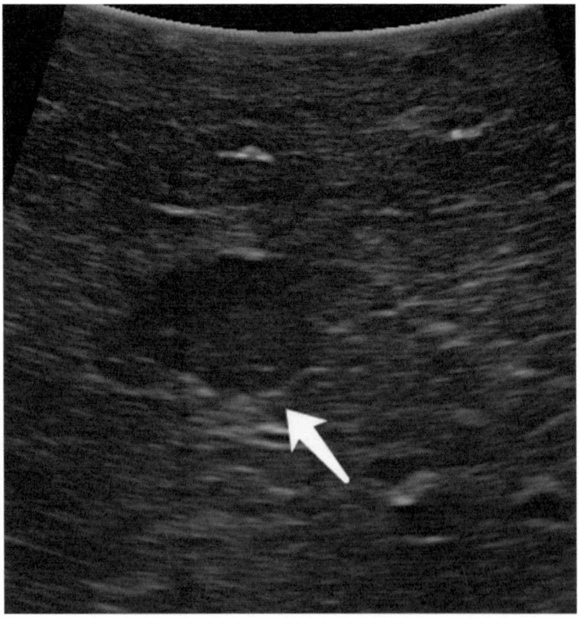

Fig. 13.8 Generally, hepatic cellular carcinoma appeared as hypo-echoic lesion (*arrow*)

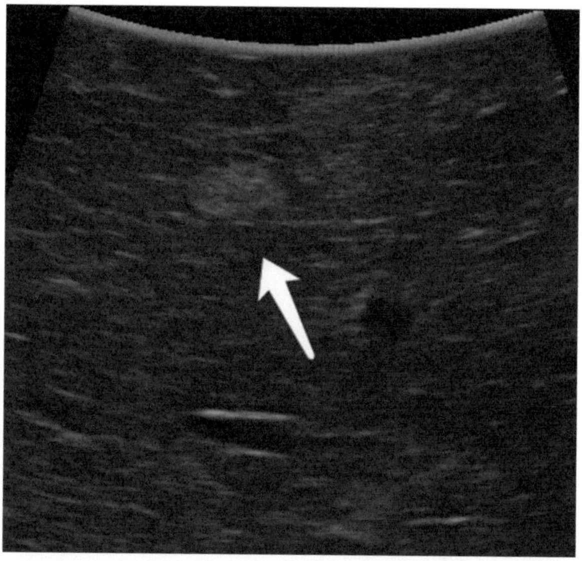

Fig. 13.9 Cirrhotic nodes appeared as hyper-echoic lesion with sharp margin which is usually smaller than 1 cm (*arrow*)

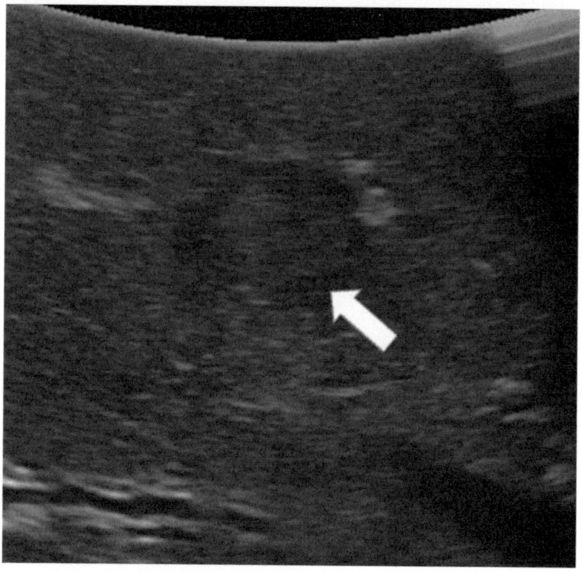

Fig. 13.10 Hepatic cellular carcinoma appeared as inhomogeneous echoic lesion (*arrow*)

1. Liver resection related complications, such as bleeding, bile leakage, and insufficient remnant hepatic function. The risk of bleeding and bile leakage of RFA assisted laparoscopic liver resection is lower than that of conventional laparoscopic liver resection.
2. Heat injury of adjacent tissue, such as gallbladder, diaphragm, and gastrointestinal tract.
3. Hepatic abscess.

4. Biliary injury.
5. Skin burn.
6. Hemoglobinuria.

13.5 Notes

1. During surgery, the coagulation area generally appeared as a hypoechoic area in ultrasonography (Figs. 13.12 and 13.13).

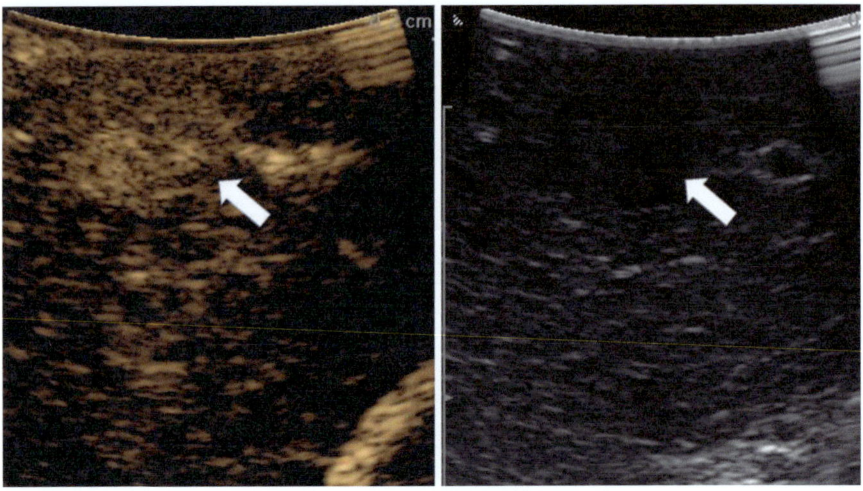

Fig. 13.11 Contrast enhanced ultrasound revealed a hyper-enhanced lesion suggesting malignancy

Fig. 13.12 Coagulation area appeared as a hypoechoic area

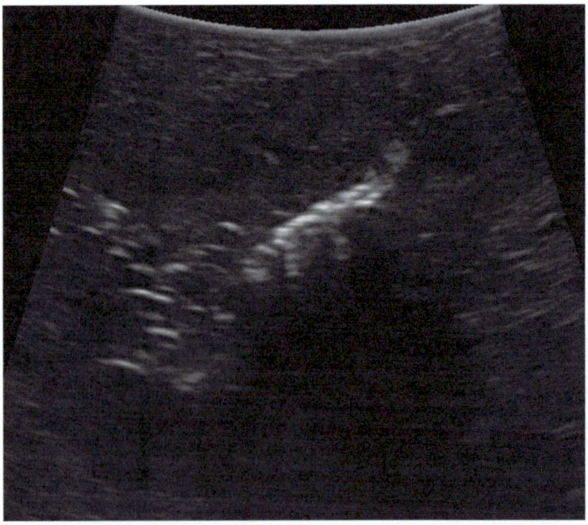

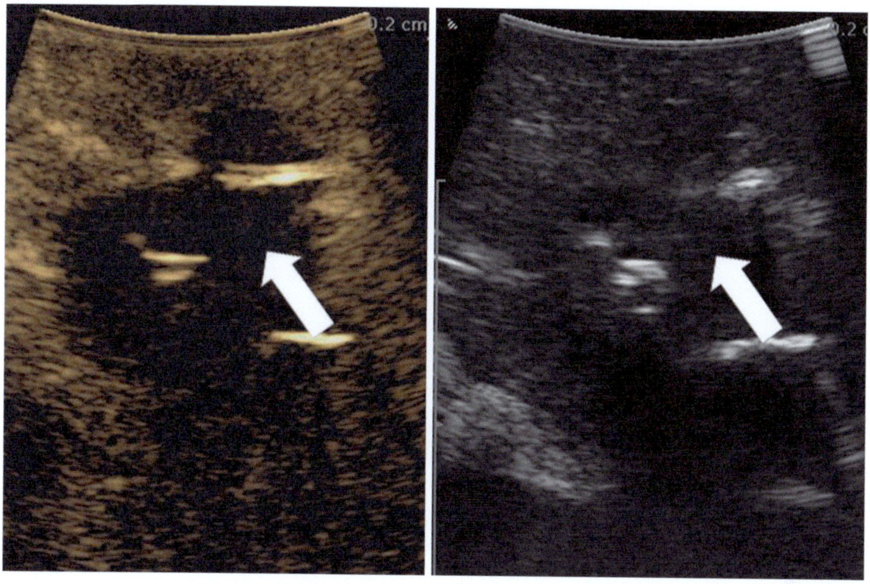

Fig. 13.13 The hypoechoic area in conventional ultrasound appeared as non-contrast enhanced area in contrast enhanced ultrasound (*arrow*)

2. The RFA assisted liver resection technique is useful for both open liver resection and laparoscopic liver resection.
3. This technique can also be used in laparoscopic regular liver resection, which can reduce the blood loss effectively.
4. The post-operative biochemistry results and the temperature should be paid attention on.

References

Pai M, et al. Liver resection with bipolar radiofrequency device: Habib™ 4X. HPB (Oxford). 2008;10(4):256–60.

Weber JC, et al. New technique for liver resection using heat coagulative necrosis. Ann Surg. 2002;236(5):560–3.

Index

R. Liu, *Laparoscopic Liver Resection*,
https://doi.org/10.1007/978-94-017-9735-1

MIX
Papier aus verantwortungsvollen Quellen
Paper from responsible sources
FSC® C105338

If you have any concerns about our products,
you can contact us on
ProductSafety@springernature.com

In case Publisher is established outside the EU,
the EU authorized representative is:
Springer Nature Customer Service Center GmbH
Europaplatz 3, 69115 Heidelberg, Germany

Printed by Libri Plureos GmbH
in Hamburg, Germany